Praise for

# Why I Walk

Kevin Klinkenberg, one of the most productive
urban thinkers around, points us toward development
that adds economic value, build community and
improves environmental performance.

—John Norquist, President and CEO of the
Congress for the New Urbanism

This is one of those books that make you smarter.
Not "book smart" but "street smart," which is appropriate
since Kevin is writing about walking and biking city streets
instead of driving them. While he talks about his own
life and experiences, he gives you areas to examine
in your own life. He has figured out a few things,
but he's not preachy about it. The book is organized
into 4 areas that are relatable to all of us and where most
of us could create some thoughtful improvements.
Don't just take Kevin's word for it—check out the
voices of other people he's included who are
living and walking in very different cities (Denver to
Miami, D.C. to Durham, and L.A. to Brooklyn).
In whatever way you define "quality of life," this book
will inspire you to consider your daily routines and rituals
and take simple, meaningful steps (pun intended)
to refresh and enrich your life.

—Dawn Taylor, Executive Director,
American Institute of Architects Kansas City

*Why I Walk* provides an insightful look into the implications of walkability upon the daily life. Kevin explores how his choice of walking impacts overall health, psyche and ultimately the pocketbook. More importantly, *Why I Walk* provides fundamental and real-world ramifications as to the implications of a walkable lifestyle. Kevin's thoughtful and personal commentary certainly has made me rethink my day-to-day transportation choices.

—Jim Potter, partner, Development Initiatives,
Kansas City MO


While it paints a less-than-flattering picture of our present culture that this book needed to be written, we're all very fortunate that it was. If you're looking for common-sense, benefit-rich reasons to get walking (or biking), you'll find them here. And your life will be better for it.

—Scott Doyon, Principal, PlaceMakers LLC


Using his day-to-day life in Savannah as a backdrop, Kevin Klinkenberg provides compelling reasons for spending more time on our own feet and for getting to know our neighborhoods better. In plain language that seamlessly combines practical experience and contemporary urban theory, *Why I Walk* details the physical, social, financial, emotional, and even professional reasons for walking whenever and wherever we can. For some readers, Klinkenberg's book might help confirm the sense that America's "car culture" is the source of many of our social and economic ills; for others, *Why I Walk* might simply be the last bit of inspiration needed to open the front door and step outside.

—Bill Dawers, editor of *Savannah Unplugged* and longtime City Talk columnist for the *Savannah Morning News*

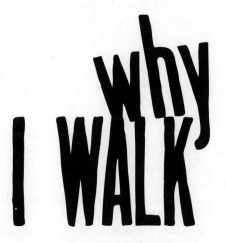

# why I WALK

## Taking a Step in the Right Direction

### Kevin Klinkenberg

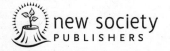

new society
PUBLISHERS

Cover design by Diane McIntosh.

Author image: from author; background image © iStock (Brian A. Jackson)

Printed in Canada. First printing June 2014.

New Society Publishers acknowledges the financial support of the Government of Canada through the Canada Book Fund (CBF) for our publishing activities.

Paperback ISBN: 978-0-86571-772-5
eISBN: 978-1-55092-569-2

Inquiries regarding requests to reprint all or part of *Why I Walk* should be addressed to New Society Publishers at the address below.

To order directly from the publishers, please call toll-free (North America) 1-800-567-6772, or order online at www.newsociety.com

Any other inquiries can be directed by mail to:

New Society Publishers
P.O. Box 189, Gabriola Island, BC V0R 1X0, Canada
(250) 247-9737

New Society Publishers' mission is to publish books that contribute in fundamental ways to building an ecologically sustainable and just society, and to do so with the least possible impact on the environment, in a manner that models this vision. We are committed to doing this not just through education, but through action. The interior pages of our bound books are printed on Forest Stewardship Council®-registered acid-free paper that is **100% post-consumer recycled** (100% old growth forest-free), processed chlorine-free, and printed with vegetable-based, low-VOC inks, with covers produced using FSC®-registered stock. New Society also works to reduce its carbon footprint, and purchases carbon offsets based on an annual audit to ensure a carbon neutral footprint. For further information, or to browse our full list of books and purchase securely, visit our website at: www.newsociety.com

Library and Archives Canada Cataloguing in Publication

Klinkenberg, Kevin, author
        Why I walk : taking a step in the right direction / Kevin Klinkenberg.

Includes index.

Issued in print and electronic formats.

ISBN 978-0-86571-772-5 (pbk.).--ISBN 978-1-55092-569-2 (ebook)

        1. Walking. 2. Walking--Economic aspects. 3. Walking--Health aspects.
4. Walking--Social aspects. I. Title.

RA781.65.K65 2014            613.7'176            C2014-902060-0
                                                                           C2014-902061-9

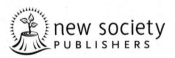

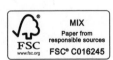

MIX
Paper from
responsible sources
FSC® C016245

# Contents

# Acknowledgments

When I finally sat down to write this book, it surprised me how quickly it spilled out on the page. But I never would have gotten to that point without the help and encouragement of so many people. While there are far too many to mention, I'd like to highlight just a few:

To my family, and especially my brother Dean. They've given me nothing but love and support over the years, and Dean's advice as a previously published author was invaluable.

To Andrea Gollin, who I first met as part of the Knight Fellowship in Community Building in Miami. Andrea walked me through editing and proofreading, and helped turn this into a real book.

To Stu Sirota & Lee Sobel, who are my regular email buddies, tough critics and lifelong pals that also met through the Knight program and the CNU.

To all of the contributors for their own personal stories – wow, I was blown away by the quality of what you all produced. Thanks for responding to my request.

To all of my friends and former co-workers in KC, especially Brian, Dan, Jerod, Katie & the whole 180 gang. You know who you are, and this wouldn't be possible without all of our efforts over the years.

To my new friends and colleagues in Savannah for opening your arms to me.

To New Society Publishers for taking a chance on my little book.

And finally, to the lovely Jamie Andersen for being so supportive of my efforts, putting up with all of the talk about it and for joining me on many great walks. We'll have many more long walks to come.

# Introduction

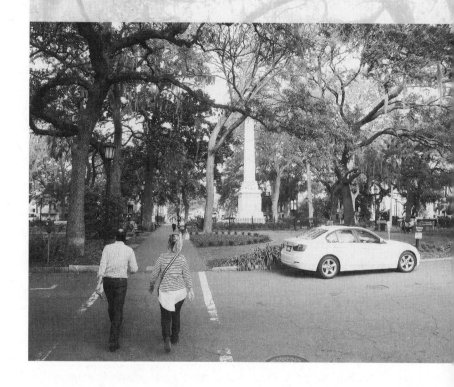

*All truly great thoughts are conceived while walking.*
— Friedrich Nietzsche, *Twilight of the Idols*

The premise of this book is very simple — I like to walk. Whether it's for a night out on the town, getting to work, running errands or even going to the grocery store, I prefer to get where I'm going using my own two feet.

For years, friends and family have regarded this choice of mine with, well, curiosity. For them and the majority of Americans, the idea of walking to a destination as opposed to driving seems rather strange.

My preference for walking has led to some interesting responses over the years:

> **Woman on date:** *"We're walking, not driving? But what shoes will I wear?"*
> **Mother:** *"You walk to that restaurant down the street? Is it safe?"*
> **Friend:** *"What do you mean you don't want a ride home? How are you going to get there?"*

Despite being viewed as something of an anomaly, not only do I continue to walk, but I find myself walking even more as the years pass. While walking is a choice that makes a lot of sense to me — for many reasons — this natural use of two legs apparently requires justification in our twenty-first century culture. After years of describing to the people in my life the many ways their own lives would improve if they would only follow in my footsteps, I decided to write this book. While in some ways this is a personal book intended to provide a look at my life that I hope is fun and informative, my larger goal is to convey the simple message that walking is a route to a much better quality of life for everyone.

My interest in walking, while largely personal, is also directly tied to my career choice. I'm an architect and urban planner and have made a career focused on creating more walkable and bike-friendly places across the country. My friends and colleagues from the world of architecture and urban planning can discuss

**JARGON ALERT:** *Walkability*

Yes, planners have coined a term for places that are best suited to walking on a regular basis. Not surprisingly, we call it *walkability*. Places that have walkability are then called *walkable communities, walkable neighborhoods* or yes, *walkable places*. All of that translates to places designed for people to navigate primarily on foot rather than primarily by driving.

in great detail the many environmental and societal benefits of walking, as can I. The list of books dealing with these topics is long and interesting, especially to planning wonks like myself. Much of the literature describes how walking can save the world.

This book is not one of those books.

This book is about how my choice to live in a walkable place and actually walking, biking and (gasp!) even riding public transportation on a daily basis benefits me — and how and why I believe it can benefit you as well. In these pages I explore the positive impact of walking on various aspects of my life including my finances, my sense of freedom, my health and my social life. Hopefully, sharing my experiences will encourage you to explore different ways of getting to your destinations.

Despite advocating for walking and walkability, by no means do I think cars are evil (as some people suggest), and everyone should immediately give up their vehicles. I own a car and have continuously owned one since I was sixteen years old. I use my car regularly for trips across town, to other towns and, of course, on the great American road trip. From an early age, my parents opened my eyes to the virtues of traveling across the country by car. Those trips and many since have been some of the best times of my life.

The difference between me and many Americans is that I do not let my car define me, nor do I want to be beholden to it. I love having the freedom to go where I want to go and do what I want to do without needing to fire up a vehicle. When it comes to transportation, I'm firmly pro-choice.

This book describes quite a bit of my daily life, which is based in Savannah, Georgia, as I write this. Those of you who are familiar with Savannah will know some of the city's wonderful qualities — including its walkability. The streets, squares and parks of the city's historic district are indeed beautiful, and among the finest in all of North America. (If you visit, please give a tip of the cap to General James Oglethorpe, who master-planned the city.) But in truth, Savannah is like many places in America. It has an old city that is compact and walkable surrounded by a vast sea of modern suburbia that is not arranged well for walking. The historic district here offers many enjoyable places to walk, but you don't need special places for your walks; you can pretty much walk anywhere. I experienced this myself when I lived in places that were much less pedestrian-friendly, and still found daily opportunities to walk. I suspect all of us can do the same.

In my particular case, I made a deliberate choice to live in Savannah. Occasionally I joke that Savannah chose me due to my love of city planning and architecture, but in truth that is not far off the mark. I moved here almost three years ago after spending the first forty years of my life in the Midwest. When the Great Recession hit, it sent a shock wave through my industry, and made an awful lot of us think about our career and life choices. For me, it created an opportunity to relocate, to start fresh. At first, I thought of it as my own (male) version of *Eat, Pray, Love,* but that quickly turned into something else entirely as I realized how much I enjoyed the city I chose.

When I thought about relocating, I considered many cities, with walkability being a requirement that was at the top of my list. Whether I looked farther south to Miami, west to Denver or Los Angeles, or even north to Chicago, I tried to imagine

**FACTOID:** *Choosing to walk and bike*

More and more young people are showing a preference for walking and biking over driving. One recent survey found that from 2001 to 2009, young people who lived in households with annual incomes of more than $70,000 increased their use of public transit by 100 percent, biking by 122 percent and walking by 37 percent.

*(Source: "Transportation and the New Generation," The Frontier Group and US PIRG Education Fund, 2012)*

which place would give me the quality of life I sought — the ability to roam freely on foot as much as possible, ride a bike comfortably and safely, and be able to afford a slower pace of life. Putting a premium on these quality-of-life factors is not unusual — it aligns me with an increasing number of people who put qualities such as a walkable, bike-friendly place at the top of their list when choosing where to live. This is especially true with the younger generation (*Generation Y* or the *Millennials*) and a little less so among *Gen X'ers* like myself.

I lived in Kansas City, Missouri, for seventeen years before moving to Savannah. Even in Kansas City, I did my best to choose a walkable lifestyle — I lived in the Midtown area — and I walked to as many destinations as I could. The going was more difficult in Kansas City than in Savannah, simply because the city isn't as well-suited to walking, but I made the best of it.

For my friends, family and colleagues in Kansas City, I hope this book answers the question they often direct my way: "Why Savannah?" And I hope it also addresses the follow-up question about when I'll move back by explaining why it's difficult for me to consider moving back to Kansas City (or anywhere that lacks these qualities, for that matter). Savannah is certainly not the only walkable city, but it's one of the best. But for the many places in our country that are not especially walkable, there is hope.

As architects and urban planners, my colleagues and I work on both existing and newly planned neighborhoods with the aim of improving our world and the lives of ordinary people. Creating better places to live can in turn improve our lives. And better places are places where we can walk.

# 1

## An Ordinary Monday

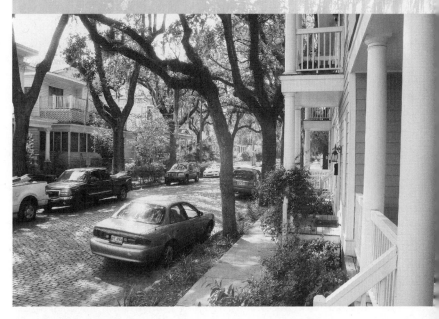

View from our stoop.

*There is this to be said for walking: it is the one method
of human locomotion by which a man or woman proceeds
erect, upright, proud and independent, not squatting on
the haunches like a frog. Little boys love machines.
Grown-up men and women like to walk.*

— Edward Abbey, *Postcards from Ed: Dispatches and
Salvos from an American Iconoclast*, 2007

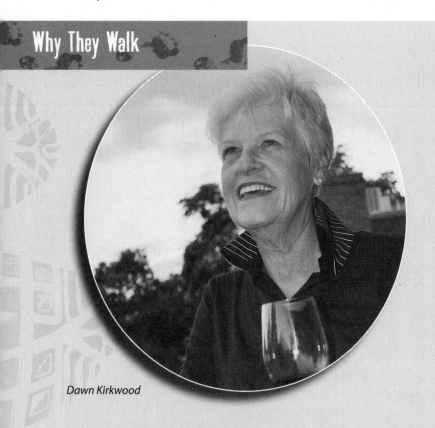

Dawn Kirkwood

I'm an independent cuss, and I make most of my life choices in support of that trait. I like having access to as many options as possible, and that includes mobility. Walking is always my first choice. I set my own pace and route. I'm out in the fresh air, I let my mind wander, and I can really look at/listen to my surroundings. I believe in doing one thing at a time, so I do not listen to music or audio books or talk on my phone while walking. It's a bit of escapism I build into my daily routine.

Since one's survival depends on being hyper-alert when biking in my city, I am not a bicycle commuter. I live near a major bike path, though, so I frequently hop on my ten-speed and peddle as fast as I can along Cherry Creek. I love that surge of power when my legs really start pumping. *That and the sense of freedom, knowing I'm completely in control, equal pure joy.*

*For practical considerations as well as sociological observations, I am a frequent user of public transit. Major bus routes and light rail stops are within walking distance of my apartment. And yes, I own a car — an '04 Toyota with 53,000 miles on the odometer.*

— Dawn Kirkwood
Denver, CO

I work from home these days. As I considered my workplace options, I also looked at sharing an office space or renting a private office. Either might work for me at some point, and I found some nice professional spaces that would be either a thirty-minute walk or a ten-minute bike ride away. That would take a bit of time, but it's honestly not that much, and it would be very enjoyable time, for the most part. But more on that later.

Some people who report to an office every day idealize working at home and think, "Wow, it must be great to have that kind of flexibility." But in actuality, working from home is not that different from going to an office or other workplace. In my twenty or so years of working in the professional world, I've worked in small offices, large office towers, my own living room, coffee shops, conference rooms and cafés. In any situation, you develop a routine and habits in order to maximize your day, and you also entertain distractions to rest and refuel. At home, I might flip on the TV at some point to take a break, whereas at work in one of my former jobs we routinely played a video game called *Redneck Rampage* whenever we could. The truth is, work is work, and we build flexibility and rigidity into our days, often without giving it much conscious thought.

But still, I'm sure my routine is different from yours. A big part of what makes my workdays distinctive is not just that I work from home, but where I live. If I lived on a typical suburban street with a cul-de-sac at the end, my daily routine would be very different. For one, it would involve a lot more driving whenever I want to leave the house. Here, most of my excursions out are walking trips. Let me walk you through (pun intended) an ordinary Monday in my life.

I roll out of bed and get cleaned up. My girlfriend Jamie rises earlier than I do, and she's kind enough to make sure there's coffee waiting downstairs. A small cup gets me started and is handy as I scan my messages and e-mails. My clients and my work span the country, so I might have e-mails from a variety of time zones to deal with at any given moment. Also, early morning is a great time for me to catch up on the news of the day, and I browse a few favorite websites that keep me abreast of what I care about. Sure, like most people, I take a look at Facebook as well.

It's not long before I've got a full belly from breakfast, and the workday is underway. At some point mid-morning, I love to take a short break and walk to my favorite coffee shop. They make a particularly great version of *café con leche*, the Cuban coffee concoction, and it puts about ten thousand watts into my veins. As the coffee shop is about a seven- or eight-minute walk

Jamie and I met shortly after I moved to Savannah. We met in large part due to a social group on Meetup.com, which used to have regular pub crawls downtown. On one fateful November evening, we pub crawled into each other at Sixpence Pub, a notorious local tavern (where Julia Roberts was filmed in the movie *Something to Talk About*). After a couple of hours of getting to know each other (and a couple of pints), the rest was history. And yes, I walked to the pub crawl, and I walked home as well. Fortunately for me, Jamie also enjoys being active and walking around the city.

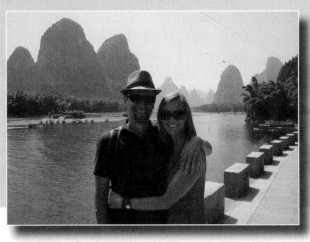

*Walk your way to love.*

away, it also gives me a chance to walk off some food and enjoy a little fresh air. On most days, I like to sit in the shop and drink the coffee, which calms down the morning work anxiety and stirs my creative juices. Some days, there's not enough time, so it's café con leche to go, and back to the laptop.

Without my quite realizing how much time has gone by, lunchtime arrives, and it's down to the kitchen to find something to eat. A lot of days lunch is something very simple in order to maximize my working time and keep my focus. On this day, I keep it light and quick so I can also get out and run a couple of errands. Today, I hop on the bicycle (my fifteen-year-old Schwinn hybrid mountain bike) and head downtown. Ten minutes later (to walk, it would take about twenty-five minutes) I'm at the post office, where I lock up the bike. From there, I'm able to walk across the street and go to the bank as well, so two important tasks are complete. Back on the bike, I head home through some beautiful streets and around tree-lined squares, feeling invigorated and ready for the afternoon. One of the beauties of this bit of errand-running is that each day I can vary my route just a little, and experience something new. Worries like traffic and parking don't even cross my mind.

Once the workday is done (which is really *never* when you work from home), it's time to do some real exercise to get my heart rate up. On this day I choose running, which is my default option. It's an easy walk of about ten minutes down to Forsyth Park, a thirty-acre city park in the midst of the neighborhood, and it's a one-mile loop around the perimeter. Today, I run three miles in the park and then run out of the park on the city sidewalks for another quarter mile or so — just to officially feel like I've done 5K. The stroll home from there is very short, but it gives me time to cool down a bit before going inside. Then it's shower, eat and get ready for the evening.

Monday nights are trivia nights when Jamie and I are in town together, and we walk over to Crystal Beer Parlor for its version of the fun. It's about a twenty-minute walk, but our route takes us through the park and some beautiful streets, so even chilly nights don't bother us much. In fact, it's often invigorating physically and mentally to stretch our legs like this in the evening. We play, and enjoy a couple beers. Valiantly, our team (Grab Something Random) competes, but we come up short of the prize money. Oh well — maybe next time. Who knew that a group of unicorns is called a *blessing*? Clearly, not us. At any rate, we stroll back home and call it a night.

All in all, it's a day filled with activities similar to a lot of other people's. I worked a full day, ate several meals, exercised and spent time with friends and loved ones. It's just that the way I went about it seems *not* so ordinary.

# 2

## Why I Walk: *Financial*

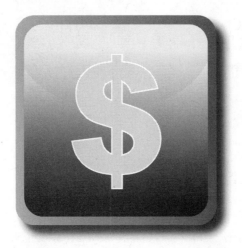

*If I could not walk far and fast,
I think I should just explode and perish.*

— Charles Dickens

## Why They Walk

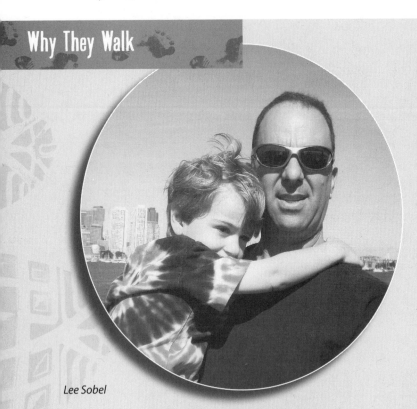

Lee Sobel

When I lived and worked in Miami, Florida, I would fill up my car two or three times a week. Then I moved to Montgomery County, Maryland, to take a job in Washington, DC. One of my housing requirements was to live near a metro station and take advantage of DC's subway. Metro is a smart way to commute. The train gave me 45 minutes of extra time each way to read, write, or simply relax. A round-trip commute, plus parking, was cheaper than driving downtown and paying for parking. Most of my weekly drive time was spent just shuttling back and forth to the Metro parking lot.

Once I got comfortable as a rail commuter, I decided to take one of the three buses in my neighborhood to the Metro station. Yes, I was saving some money by not paying for parking, but I really started riding the bus because the opportunity was there. I wasn't losing commute time by bus. And I made a personal decision to use the infrastructure my tax dollars were investing in. I never considered riding a bus in Miami for all the reasons suburbanites don't and won't ride a bus if they don't have to. Now my drive time was further reduced, mostly for weekend errands.

Then one spring I did something unexpected, I rode my bike to the Metro station. It was incredibly fun, but it wasn't enough for me. I started biking to work. First one way on alternative days, then full round-trip commutes every day. Goodbye car! Goodbye subway costs! Goodbye 20 extra pounds! Now I only drive a few times a month.

For the past two years, biking has been the primary way I commute to work. I joined DC's bikesharing program last year. During the day, I try to make bikeshare my first means of travel when going to meetings, lunches, and events. Depending on the weather, my business schedule or my family plans, I can commute to work by bike, bus or drive to the Metro. I have options and choices about how to get around that I never had in Miami. I'm not biking to save money or the environment, or to be healthy (though these are additional benefits of course). I bike because it's fun and easy. And it's fun and easy because I live in a place that provides the infrastructure and facilities to make such a choice safe and available.

— Lee Sobel
Washington, DC

As individuals and a society, we are slaves to the eighteen percent.

I speak not of the wealthy versus the poor, but of our own budgets and how much we spend just getting around.

One of the statistics about our spending that surprises people is that the average American household spends eighteen percent of its after-tax budget on transportation. That's second only to housing. Food comes in at twelve percent and health care at six percent (this, according to the US Department of Labor). Just consider that for a minute — we spend three times more on transportation than on our own health (see the sidebar "American Household Spending").

With all the political discussion given over to health care at the national level, would you have expected it to be such a relatively small part of the average American's budget? Yet, how much airtime do we give to the vast amount more we spend getting around? Will we ever see a presidential debate focused on transportation?

Walking saves me a lot of money.

Why do we pay so much for transportation?

Very simply, it's because we are dependent on our cars to get us around. That's why planners and urban designers like me use the phrase "auto-dependent" when referring to many of our cities and suburbs. In far too many places, it's difficult, if not impossible, to attend to the daily business of life unless you are driving.

Digging deeper into the numbers, the AAA's latest estimates have the cost of owning a mid-size car at $9,519 per year (calculated for an average of fifteen thousand miles). That number factors in all the costs involved — average car payment, insurance, taxes, gas, maintenance, etc. Drive a bigger car, or more miles, and the cost goes up.

# American Household Spending

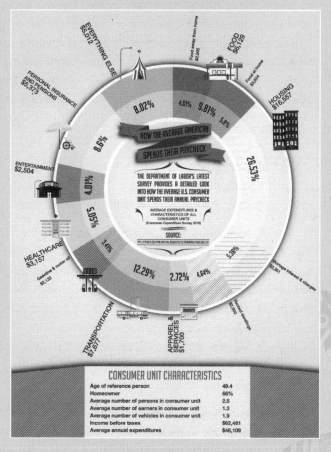

http://visualeconomics.creditloan.com/how-the-average-us-consumer-spends-their-paycheck/
(Source: Department of Labor, 2010)

Note: The transportation statistics shown here are averages. Newer studies are showing that in many suburban parts of the country, the true cost of transportation is much higher, upward of thirty to forty percent of after-tax income.

(Source: "H+T Affordability Index," Center for Neighborhood Technology, www.cnt.org)

By contrast, the cost of walking is a pair of shoes. The cost of biking is a few hundred bucks a year for most riders. The cost of taking public transit is several hundred dollars (depending on your city). But still, it's a fraction of the price of car ownership.

It's a great exercise to run the numbers on your own situation. I currently don't have a car payment, and my car is about seven years old. Averaged over the last two years, I've driven about ten thousand miles per year and my expenses are:

> Insurance: $100/month
> Gas: $167/month
> Taxes & Fees: $13/month
> Service: $40/month
> *Total: $320/month, or about $3,840 per year*

So, I spend about forty percent of the average cost for driving. Plus, I should note that my gas costs have come down dramatically in the last twelve months due to less long-distance road tripping. As a result of my lifestyle choices, I have an extra five to six thousand dollars per year in my pocket compared to the average American. Not too shabby.

Here's another exercise. Suppose my car needs to be replaced, and I have to make payments on a new vehicle. How does that affect my budget?

> Car payment: $350/month (average new car, five-year loan)
> Insurance: $150/month (newer car)
> Gas: $100/month (slightly more fuel efficient and 8,000 miles per year)
> Taxes: $20/month (newer car)
> Service: $10/month (only basic maintenance)
> *Total: $630/month, or about $7,560 per year*

Those totals are still two thousand dollars less than the AAA's averages, even with a new car payment. When you start to run these numbers for yourself, you quickly see that the biggest immediate savings when driving less are on gas and repairs. That much is obvious. In addition, reduced driving translates to less need for fuel and less wear and tear on the vehicle.

But the most significant savings are found elsewhere. In fact, they are in the next section of this chapter.

I'm under no illusions that we can all suddenly ditch our cars and walk everywhere. As I noted earlier, too many of our communities are not set up for that today. Many people have no choice but to drive to work, sometimes very long distances. But what if you could reduce your car use and walk, bike or take transit more? If you own one car, you likely can't eliminate it, but by making some changes, you could pretty easily save $4,000 to $5,000 per year. What would you do with an extra $4,000 in your pocket?

**JARGON ALERT: *Transit.***

Yes, I'm basically talking about the bus. Some cities are lucky enough to have a viable subway, light rail or elevated rail system, but for most places the public transportation alternative is the bus.

If you live in a multiple car household, what would happen if you could eliminate one car? Now you're talking potential savings of ten thousand dollars per year. How would that impact your savings or your budget for that vacation you really want to take? More on this, later in this chapter.

The bottom line is this: one major reason I like to walk is *it saves me a lot of money.*

My car lasts longer, saving me even more money.

It's an obvious point, isn't it? If you drive about five thousand miles per year instead of fifteen thousand miles per year, your car will last longer and you will save money in the long run. That's why I like to think of the money-savings for walking in these terms:

*Big savings:  gas and repairs*
*Biggest savings:  car lasts longer, so I go without a payment for*
                          *more years*

Let's explore this a bit.

The previous section reviewed the average costs of car ownership and outlined a description of my current situation. Note that the average costs cited include a car payment and service as major components; without those two items, the cost would certainly be less than AAA's estimate of $9,519 per year.

So what additional financial effect does increased walking and biking have versus driving?

AAA estimates an average of fifteen thousand miles per year for car use. Over the course of a typical five-year car loan, that car reaches seventy-five thousand miles, assuming it started with zero. In most cases, it's likely to be more than that since cars rarely are purchased with zero miles. At that level of mileage, a car starts to need some very expensive repairs (which is why warranties typically expire around or before then). All parts on cars eventually need replacement, whether they be tires, brakes, belts, shocks, head gaskets and on and on. The more use the parts have, the sooner they need replacement.

But what if you drive only five thousand miles per year instead of fifteen thousand? At the end of a five-year car loan, you'd have a vehicle with twenty-five thousand miles on it — if you bought it new. But even if you bought it used, with ten thousand miles on it to start, your car would have still only have about thirty-five thousand miles. A car with that relatively low mileage is a long way from requiring the more expensive maintenance. And most importantly, that car is a very long way from needing to be replaced.

## A Few of the More Costly and Typical Automobile Maintenance Expenses

- Timing belts every sixty thousand or ninety thousand miles
- Front brakes every twenty thousand to thirty thousand miles
- Rear brakes every sixty thousand miles
- Transmission service every sixty thousand miles
- Tires vary widely, but often every twenty-five thousand to fifty thousand miles
- Spark plugs every thirty thousand to sixty thousand miles
- Distributor cap and rotor every sixty thousand miles

*(Source: http: www.autorepairadvisors.com/a_list_of_normal_maintenance_ite.shtml.* This is just one source; there are numerous websites and owner's manuals to be found online that offer advice on routine maintenance.)

While the owner who drives a car fifteen thousand miles per year might be frugal and stretch the car for another five years past the car loan payoff, the owner who drives five thousand miles per year could conceivably have it payment-free for ten or even fifteen more years. This is where the big savings really kick in. With much-reduced driving, you can still own a car, and own it without a payment for a very long period of time.

When I look at these numbers, I see a few key advantages to lower car mileage. First, there's the obvious benefit of lower monthly costs, as I outlined in the previous section. Second, the savings allow you to squirrel away a small amount of money each month (perhaps $50) to allocate toward eventually replacing the car. That money doesn't add up to much if you only drive a car for a year or two beyond the end of the loan, but if you have the car for five, seven or ten years after the loan, that small amount

## Is five thousand miles per year really possible?

That's about four hundred miles per month, or about one hundred miles per week. In my case, it is very easy to keep mileage down to five thousand miles annually — sometimes, it's even less. I typically only use my car in town for some shopping trips and a few recreational outings (the beach, the movies). Those trips add up to about fifty miles per week. Since I live in a walkable location, I have the option to walk, bike or ride the bus to work as well, so I don't need my car for that. It's the long-distance trips (road trips) that cause my mileage to reach a higher number, but even with those, I estimate that I'll put only five thousand miles on my car each year going forward.

will add up to anywhere from $3,000 to $6,000 toward a new vehicle. And, of course, paying more up front means a substantially reduced monthly payment for the new car.

This is what economists call a *virtuous circle*. Walking more and driving less pays you back more and more over time.

## I am unconcerned with gas prices.

The price of gas is constantly in our faces. It's the one thing we buy that we're reminded of on a daily basis, since the price is always displayed outside in large print. Some might say we're obsessed with gas costs.

Gas (and oil) prices dominate the news, our politics, and even our national mood at times. When the price of gas rises substantially, as it did in 2008, it sends us into a mild panic. When the prices drop, we perk up and think of hitting the open road. This instability and uncertainty puts many of our wallets and moods on a constant roller coaster.

**Make Walking & Biking Easy Tip 1:**
*Use the Front Door*

One of the first and easiest steps you can take is simply using the front door regularly instead of a back or garage door. Getting in the habit of entering and exiting your home or apartment in this manner subtly makes you prioritize walking instead of using the car.

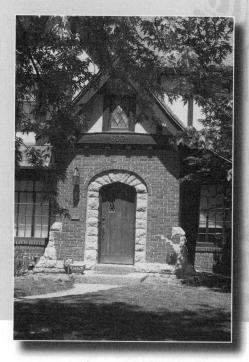

For me, gas prices are pretty irrelevant. Since I get around primarily without driving, I don't fill my tank up regularly enough to really give gas prices much thought.

For the average driver, at fifteen thousand miles per year, it's quite the opposite. A weekly fill-up is a given, if not two or three times per week, depending on the vehicle and gas mileage. Understandably, that frequency at the pump makes people very aware of price swings. An average increase of fifty cents per gallon over the course of the year could cost a driver several hundred dollars more per year.

But when you're a walker or a bicyclist, even dramatic increases have very little direct effect on your pocketbook. Of course, since we rely so much on trucking for goods and services, gas costs do impact all of us indirectly.

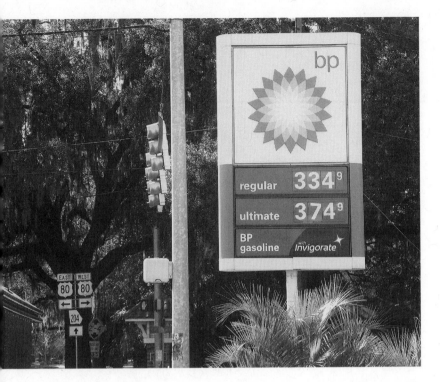

*Our national obsession.*

While we can't control all costs, what we *can* control is how we choose to live and get around. If I keep to a goal of about five thousand miles per year, an increase in the price of a gallon of gas by fifty cents or even one dollar in a year only affects me to the tune of around one hundred dollars. That's about two dollars per week, or about a cup of coffee. That's a small enough amount that I barely notice. If my car were a more fuel-efficient model, I would sense it to an even lesser degree.

Can you imagine how it would impact our culture and our politics if all of us were so unconcerned with the price of oil and gas? What else would we have to talk about?

Your choice: stress about gas prices all you want. Or join me for a walk, and enjoy life a bit more.

Spending less on transportation allows me more freedom with my money.

*Save money, live better!* No, this is not an infomercial.

What would happen to our ability to pay for other items in our budgets if we cut our transportation expenses in half (which, incidentally, would still leave us spending more on transportation than we do on health care)?

As I've considered my budget and lifestyle over the last several years, I've realized the opportunities that increased walking creates. Walking potentially benefits me in three very different ways financially:

- I can save more money for a rainy day.
- I can live just as well on a smaller salary.
- I can spend more money on things that make life happier for me — more travel, more entertainment or even a nicer home.

Saving for a rainy day is a great goal. But how often do we follow through? Do any of us sock away enough for the future? The truth is, any way we can find to save a few bucks and keep more in the bank is a good thing. Whether it adds up to a few hundred dollars or a few thousand, with the time value of money, we can all be a little more secure and prepared for life's curve balls by saving more.

Looking at our financial situation from another perspective, how much more easily could each of us maintain our current standard of living on a reduced income by cutting back on certain large expenses, like transportation? This is certainly an approach that's worked well for me. Reducing household expenses has an amazing ability to provide for less stress, more leisure time and more disposable income.

We often talk about downsizing as a means toward living a simpler life, with fewer "things" and thus decreased expenses. Instead, we can simply change our means of transportation and achieve many of the same goals. With less money going out, we feel less pressure to constantly make more, so there is less of the associated job stress that comes with the chase. With less time spent in cars and in traffic, we might find more leisure time and social time (more on that later). While we often think of money in terms of the things it can buy for us, in order to enhance our lives, we can shift to thinking of the many good things that come from needing to spend less money thanks to our choices.

If spending *less* isn't convincing, then why not think of all the other things you could spend *more* money on if you had four, five or ten thousand extra dollars in your pocket. How about that overseas vacation? Done. Want to eat out an extra night per week? Done. Maybe you prefer to buy a larger home, or have nicer stuff in it? Done. Maybe you just want to pay off your

## How Can You Spend Your Savings?

Here are some ideas (approximate cost per person):

- One week vacation to Paris: $3,000
- Long weekend beach getaway in Mexico: $1,500
- Eating out once per week for a year, nice restaurant: $2,000
- Mortgage cost per year for an extra $50,000 of house improvements: $3,600
- New living room furniture and big-screen TV with sur-round sound: $3,500

This is what walking can do for your life. It can allow you to spend money where you really want to spend it, instead of on something that gets you from point A to point B.

credit cards or spend more on shoes. You can do any of those things and more by spending less in the one area in which, I would argue, we routinely overspend.

## Walking is good for my career.

The next three sections of this chapter deal with financial considerations that are more indirect than direct. These factors still impact my life, but not in the same way that filling up a gas tank every month directly affects my budget. These considerations are more about the indirect financial benefits of choosing to live in a walkable place.

First, walking around more has a beneficial impact on my professional life.

You may be thinking: How can that be?

The answer is really quite simple when you think about it. When I walk more often, I have more face-to-face encounters with other people. I run into people (sometimes literally) on the sidewalk, in stores I might pop in and out of, or en route to a destination. These interactions are in marked contrast to driving, where I only encounter people as obstacles to where I am going.

But how do these interactions impact my career?

I believe the simple cliché is true: it's not what you know, it's who you know. The more we expand the circles of human connections, the more people we know. As we encounter people repeatedly, we get to know them better, and relationships deepen. Many of these interactions will ultimately spark connections, ideas or opportunities — they are a form of networking, which is a critical part of any person's or business's success.

Living in a walkable place, or just walking more often, makes for far more chance encounters and, well, just far more encounters. When we drive, we are sealed off from other humans, despite our cell phones and other advanced technology. It may not seem like a big deal, but an hour a day walking instead of an hour a day driving adds up to two weeks per year of time — two weeks in which we can potentially meet others and have conversations that enhance our career potential.

In his book *The Rise of the Creative Class,* Richard Florida explains that people in creative industries tend to cluster in walkable, diverse places and that cities need to plan for this as part of their economic development.

The reason that creative industries in particular like to be clustered together in walkable places is because of the encounters I'm discussing — in these places, there is a greater potential for interaction with people of the same or different professions, which sparks thinking and, ultimately, innovation.

But the professional benefits of walking don't apply only to those in creative industries. If you're in a service industry, the benefits are no different. The extra encounters with people walking around are chances to essentially market yourself and/or your business. We don't think of it that way, but it is an aspect of our interactions. This is a conversation I've had more than once with a server from a local restaurant or bar when running into them around town:

> **Server:** "Hey, how's it going?"
>
> **Me:** *"Great, thanks. Been busy lately?"*
>
> **Server:** *"Yeah, in fact I'm working tomorrow night. We have a great band playing. You should come by!"*
>
> **Me:** *"Definitely — I'll come by and check it out."*
>
> **Server:** *"Fantastic, see you then!"*

That simple exchange is the kind of friendly, daily thing that happens easily when I walk, but simply does not happen when driving. If I do show up, the server puts some additional income in her pocket, and it benefits the owner as well.

Simply following logic, more interaction leads to more and better contacts. More and better contacts lead to more opportunities. More opportunities lead to better prospects for my career. Yes, walking more can indeed help my career and income, and yours as well.

> **If I choose to own property, owning in a walkable neighborhood is a wise investment.**

I saw the movie *Enron: The Smartest Guys in the Room* a few years back; it told the story of the rise and fall of the infamous energy corporation. While it was a fascinating tale of manipulation and corruption in corporate America, it was also a very sad tale for thousands of Enron employees. It wasn't so much the jobs lost that was sad (though that was obviously a tragedy), but how so many people had invested their entire retirement portfolio in Enron stock and lost it all when the company collapsed.

The story really resonated with what investment advisors routinely tell me: diversify your portfolio. With a diverse portfolio, I will likely not have huge runs up in value, but am protected against a huge losses should some of it go down the drain.

There's a similarly troublesome practice in the world of agriculture. When certain crops become profitable, farmers have historically rushed to plant that crop to cash in on the rise in price of that commodity. When that happens, it often opens up the crop to vulnerability of attack — a particular bug, disease or weather pattern can quickly wipe out an entire year's worth of income since there is less diversity in the landscape. This monocultural approach largely created the Dust Bowl in the 1930s and is one of the ongoing threats of industrial agriculture.

Ignoring the need for diversity in stocks and in agriculture is essentially the same tactic — it is a high-risk, short-term gamble for getting rich quick. In some cases, it works out. But in most cases, it fails spectacularly.

Similarly, lack of diversity in real estate is risky. It's so pervasive that we almost don't notice anymore, and we've actually been led to believe that it's a smart investment of our housing dollars. I'm referring here to neighborhoods or subdivisions in which the houses are all essentially the same.

For many years, the accepted wisdom in real estate has been to own a home that is roughly similar to the other homes in the neighborhood — not too much nicer, not too much less expensive. That strategy has been thought of as the least risky approach, especially when it comes time to sell the house.

The problem with this line of thinking is that when neighborhoods lack diversity in housing, they become highly vulnerable to change, much like those single-crop fields. While a house may be a family's biggest investment, housing is still a consumer product and subject to the whims of the marketplace. As humans consume, we frequently change our minds about what kinds of homes and locations are desirable. One year it might be all about single-story homes with a master bedroom down and a walk-out basement; a couple of years later, and all the rage could shift to traditional two stories with all the bedrooms up. There are also the variables of school district desirability, proximity to work places and retail, and even construction quality. The point is, any situation where all of the homes are very similar is inherently fragile. Your best bet from an investment standpoint is to get in and out quickly.

Buying in a walkable place is a wiser long-term investment because walkable neighborhoods are by nature more diverse. Any good walkable neighborhood will contain a wide mixture of types of houses and apartments, alongside nearby businesses, churches and public buildings. This mixture gives a place interest and makes it appealing to walk through. But it also has the side effect of warding off dramatic price declines, since it appeals to — as people in the business like to say — a variety of market segments.

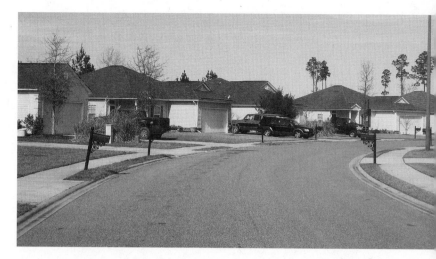

*Too much of the same thing is not a good thing.*

In a walkable neighborhood, if a certain type of house on the street becomes unfashionable or a property goes into disrepair, it won't harm the whole street. The first house I owned was on a street that was generally very nice, but it always had at least one or two houses that looked pretty bad. But the sheer variety of size and style of the other houses meant these were isolated cases. By contrast, in a neighborhood of like houses, whole streets can turn from good to lousy in just a few years when that particular type of house becomes less desirable. Think about all those cracker-box houses built in the years immediately after World War II. Practically every city in the country has at least one entire area populated with those homes. They were fine enough as housing for the generation returning from the war, but within a couple of decades, the houses were considered small and out of fashion. As that happened, entire subdivisions and streets lost their value, and we heard the first cries calling for suburban re-development. Many such places have been in decline ever since.

Life contains no guarantees, but owning real estate in a walkable, diverse neighborhood can be a key element to a balanced

## Walkscore and Housing Value

You may have heard of a cool website called Walkscore (or maybe you haven't). It rates an address based on how walkable it is. Walkscore.com is the Internet address, and it's easy to plug your own residence in to see how it rates. More interesting were the results of a study that the organization CEO for Cities did, which showed that increased walks-core directly translates to increased home value. Check it out: http://blog.walkscore.com/wp-content/uploads/2009/08/WalkingTheWalk_CEOsforCities.pdf.

investment portfolio by protecting against significant declines in value. How important is that diversity? Just ask the folks who used to work for Enron.

**I don't have to pay an HOA to maintain my streets and public spaces.**

OK, granted, this is in part because I live in an older neighborhood that was built long before Home Owners Associations (HOAs) became common.

But still, it's a real benefit to me. Hear me out on this one.

I know that some people really like living in a neighborhood where a small group of nosy neighbors collect money from the residents each month, argue about how to spend it, and hire their own trash services. I don't. I find it obnoxious — something that belongs in the realm of city government.

Believe me, I understand the frustration some people have when it comes to working with city government. My profession and my civic endeavors have resulted in countless hours spent working with innumerable departments in city halls around the country. Some of my experiences were surprisingly good. Some were not. But is trying to work with the city really any worse than neighborhood politics and all the petty arguments that ensue?

Allow me to back up for a minute. Why do we even have HOAs?

While an historical analysis would likely reveal several factors explaining why HOAs developed and became so predominant, the primary reason they came to be was to pick up the slack for cities that weren't performing basic services. The residents in many upscale neighborhoods were happy to spend a little more money to make sure the trash was picked up, the parks clean, and the grass mowed along the street.

But I'd submit that, over time, cities have improved in terms of these basic services and are more responsive to residents. Additionally, these services are already part of municipal tax bills, and I don't really enjoy paying twice for basic services.

What does all this have to do with walking?

Walkable places by nature are more compact. In order for walkable neighborhoods to work their best, destinations need to be close by so that walking can be viable and enjoyable. This compactness tends to mean more people live in the same area per square mile than they do in places designed for driving.

That density has a great spin-off benefit for the provision of city services and the people who live there. Because the neighborhoods are more compact, they are more efficient to serve per person, and cities can afford to do more.

### FACTOID: *Home Owners Associations*
HOAs had their beginnings in the late nineteenth and early twentieth centuries, but didn't become widespread until the 1960s. Today, about one in five Americans is governed by an HOA, according to a 2010 estimate by the Community Associations Institute.

# Why One Developer Decided Against Setting up an HOA

R. John Anderson and his partners developed the walkable Doe Mill neighborhood in Chico, California, starting in 2001. Here he explains why he chose not to set up an HOA for the two hundred-plus homes in the development:

> I looked really hard at the best older neighborhoods in Chico, California, and Saint Paul, Minnesota, at both the hardware of the built place and the social software of how people interacted. I thought a lot about the stuff that adds up to make places and the interactions between people better and at the stuff that erodes a place and the connections between people.
>
> The development standards and zoning of Chico interfered with our ability to build a walkable neighborhood like the city's own Mansion Park or The Streets, but the day-to-day governance that the city provided for those older neighborhoods seemed to work pretty well for the people who live there today. What would an HOA actually add to the lives of the people who were going to live in the Doe Mill neighborhood?
>
> The HOAs operating in the conventional subdivisions in town seem to do only a mediocre job of taking care of common facilities, are a source of petty politics for the residents, and present residents with a monthly bill for something that the folks who live in the older neighborhoods get as part of the city's typical basic services.
>
> HOAs are about agreeing to abide by a contract, knowing that disputes will be settled by the threat of liens and litigation. That seems like moving away from

the idea of figuring out how to get along with your neighbors; instead it's eroding civility with a very conditional agreement to be civil. There is not much poetry or hope in a prenuptial agreement, and HOA documents read like prenups. I didn't want to invest our efforts in a cynical work-around, and I didn't think it was fair to get others to sign up for it.

— R. John Anderson
Chico, California

When I lived in Kansas City, I had an interesting exchange with my Public Works director. I wrote to complain about the lack of some basic services in my neighborhood, such as street sweeping. My point of comparison to him was my brother's neighborhood in St. Louis, which had the streets cleaned every week.

After an exchange of several polite and informative letters, he finally got to the crux of the matter. Because Kansas City is so spread out (1,460 people per square mile) compared to St. Louis (4,805 people per square mile), it simply cannot afford to provide the same level of services.

I should note that St. Louis is a city that had been losing population for decades. It now has only one-third of the population it had in 1950. Yet even with that significant of a population decrease, due to its compact nature, St. Louis is able to provide better cleaning, trash and recycling pickup, cheaper water and more. Why? Because it was originally built as a compact and mostly walkable city. St. Louisans would likely argue it's lost quite a bit of that over the years, and I would tend to agree.

But the basic point remains. If a city or neighborhood is walkable and therefore compact, it can better afford to provide basic services. For my own selfish benefit, that means I don't have to pay an additional "tax" to an HOA to get these things done.

# Why They Walk

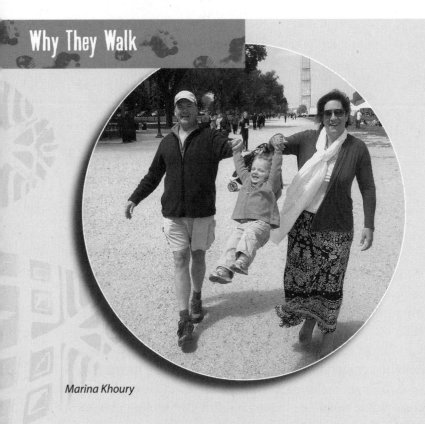

Marina Khoury

*I recently moved from one great city to another: Miami to the DC metro area, but my life here feels nobler and distinctly richer. I currently live in Lakelands, work in Kentlands, and every day, I am gratified to see these new towns function exactly the way they are intended to. I have dedicated my professional life to designing vibrant communities and adding vitality to neighborhoods. And walking, or the elegant, safe and always interesting possibility walking brings, is one of the greatest contributors to that happy success.*

*I can extol the virtues of walking all day, and its many tangible benefits are well documented. I know it is better for the environment simply because it decreases my personal carbon emissions. I know it is better for my physical health and emotional well-being as it not* only decreases my chances of obesity-related diseases, but it actually promotes happiness. I am all for that! I can attest to the fact that it is a financial boon for my wallet as these two walkable communities perform better economically and command significantly higher premiums in housing values than the sprawl that surrounds them. These are all worthy rewards, but it is a walk's intangible benefits that are even more compelling.

As seasons evolve and time flows, so does my experience of walking. I am the mother of an active eighteen-month-old daughter, Lyla, who absolutely delights in being outdoors, regardless of the weather. So we go on walks to parks, to explore and discover or to spend time in an activity we both enjoy, separately but together. We see the world differently, partly because she is happily discovering it for the first time. Personally, as an architect, I enjoy the casual study of the buildings I stroll by, and walking gives me the feel and understanding of the character of a place like nothing else can. But as a twin, I thrive on human contact and chance encounters that keep me connected to my community. I chat easily, if briefly, with many neighbors, whether in their garden, on their porch or on the sidewalk. I notice the new couple strolling hand in hand, oblivious of anything but each other. I smile at the teenage skateboarders who have willfully taken over the street, even if temporarily. Sometimes these walks are meditative and have a way of calming me and clearing my head. My husband and I have solved plenty of challenges, as ideas somehow come easier when strolling. As Henry David Thoreau eloquently said, "the moment my legs begin to move, my thoughts begin to flow." How true.

As we walk, I notice the usual while Lyla notices things within her height. Walking is her great adventure, and she is truly experiencing the sidewalks as her own personal outdoor playroom. It is a joy to watch the world reveal itself to her in this manner. She squeals with delight as she notices the ladybug crawling on the colorful flowerbed we pass or as she haplessly chases the squirrel she glimpsed at the base of the tree. She boldly attempts to pat each and every dog we stroll by. She tap dances around the paving patterns etched in the plaza. She has made plenty of new friends while out on walks while providing me with yet another good excuse to humbly do so as well. So much flows from our precious walks together, and I want to keep enjoying them for as long as I can, because I know this carefree and innocent time will pass. And then it will be on to the next compelling reason to keep on walking, hopefully always with Lyla, for the rest of my life.

— Marina Khoury
Gaithersburg, MD

# 1ˢᵗ Interlude — *An amble to necessary places*

Some places are staples of our daily or weekly existence. Here's a few of mine that I walk to.

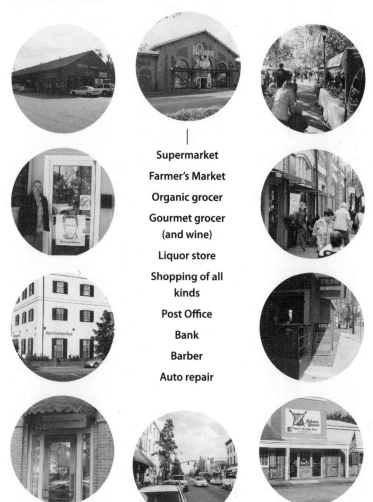

Supermarket

Farmer's Market

Organic grocer

Gourmet grocer
(and wine)

Liquor store

Shopping of all
kinds

Post Office

Bank

Barber

Auto repair

*Walking in the morning takes you to beautiful places where
light and shade make love.*

— Mohamed Shareef

# 3

## Why I Walk: *Freedom*

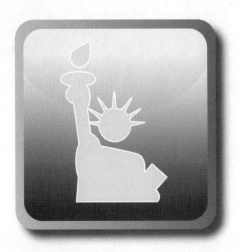

For (Jane Austen and the readers of Pride and Prejudice),
as for Mr. Darcy, Elizabeth Bennett's solitary walks express
the independence that literally takes the heroine out of the
social sphere of the houses and their inhabitants, into a
larger, lonelier world where she is free to think: walking
articulates both physical and mental freedom.

— Rebecca Solnit, *Wanderlust: A History of Walking*

## Why They Walk

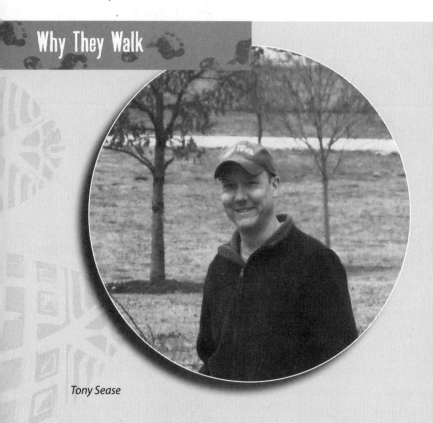

Tony Sease

The Danish architect Jan Gehl notes that "Life takes place on foot." I think about that observation often. So when asked why I walk, one simple reply is, "I walk to live." For food, for health, for work, for fun. What does my walking life look like? First, there is food. And second, there is food. And then, there is more food. Whether from family, the Farmer's Market, summer music at Brightleaf or American Tobacco, or multiple walks per week to the local Whole Foods, every journey somehow seems to involve food (even the pre-school commute, unless my son is riding his bike, fits this pattern, as it includes bananas, goldfish crackers or raisins).

With two children under four, any trip taken without buckling a toddler into the confines of a car seat is a victory. So every Saturday *of the year, when in town, we walk. Every day, in fact, we walk, but Saturdays are special because for nearly nine months of the year we walk to the downtown Farmer's Market, a veritable social hub of our city a mile from our home. The other months, the market doesn't open until ten, so we make a beeline instead for the downtown bakeries. The Farmer's Market is a weekly civic festival complete with sidewalk musicians (Andy the violin player is our son's favorite); crafts; playground features like the modernist reinterpretation of Noah's Ark, the concrete turtle and cardinal, and the steel truss bridge over the stream; and fresh vegetables and fruits, organic meats, eggs from over a dozen farms — nothing from more than fifty miles away. Locally roasted coffee, locally brewed beer in growlers, and there are the baked goods, too, all local. Mostly, though, there are the people, familiar faces from all walks of life congregating for food, fun, volunteering, or simply for homemade donuts.*

*We walk past half a dozen coffee shops along the way, opting for amazing macchiatos and fresh beignets at one, or specials like lemon chess pie and buttermilk donuts at another. Typical of the social web of walking, we know the owners of both shops. My wife went to high school with one and delivered the other's first child nearly a decade ago.*

*Walking, though, is not just on weekends. We walk the kids to their preschool, passing their future elementary school along the way. We walk to the corner store, for our seemingly daily gallon of milk. We walk to work. We walk to the grandparents' house. We walk a block to campus, for teaching, for reading, for playing on the grass lawns. I have walked to basketball games at Cameron Indoor, to football games at Wallace Wade and to Durham Bulls games. We walk to dinner frequently, and in the summer we walk to music in the courtyard at Brightleaf — much more of a cross-section of Durham life than even the Farmer's Market. It's at the Brightleaf events, perhaps more than others, that it's apparent that so few have the option of walking all the places we are able. And so many miss out on the daily interactions, the culinary, caffeinatory, educational, recreational, cultural — and happenstance — joys of daily walking. So much remains to be done in order for life to take place on foot.*

— Tony Sease
Durham, NC

From the beginning of the car age, cars have been marketed to us as tickets to freedom. In our own cars, we can choose our individual path and get to our destination quickly, unimpeded by the inconvenience/lack of speed of walking or public transportation. There is no point in denying the truth of that scenario — all things being equal, getting in a car affords tremendous mobility. In a car, not only are we not limited to destinations reachable only by foot, bike, bus or train, but cars allow us to choose our own route and set our own schedule.

The problem, however, is that all things are no longer equal. Car ownership began to become ubiquitous in the 1950s. Since then, we have revolutionized the ways in which our cities are planned and built. Caught up in the allure of the car age, we remade our places, and built new ones, that cater to cars. Today we often forget that prior to World War II, every city in America was built for easy walking and biking. In fact, the idea of living in a walkable place is nothing radical. What was radical was the program we undertook to build an entirely new type of human life. We built networks of roadways and freeways like nothing any society had ever seen before. We tore down entire neighborhoods to accommodate these roads as well as the parking lots and garages required by the cars that would travel these roads; at the same time, we ripped out the tracks for streetcars and trains.

As we became drunk on cars and the modern age, we forgot some basic things about human nature. One of our core characteristics is that we crave freedom and choices.

I have more freedom because I live in a walkable neighborhood.

Writing this book in 2013 and looking back several decades, it's apparent that our society has come full circle in terms of the freedom of mobility. Where the car once provided freedom from the crowded, old city, it now is a device that enslaves us. Yes, I do mean enslaved.

Like many people my age and younger, when I was growing up, we used a car to get around everywhere; I was barely aware that there was any way to live that wasn't entirely car reliant. For about three generations now, Americans have grown up fully immersed in the car culture, not knowing alternatives — and that's a problem.

The problem, at its most basic, is that we have become dependent on cars. While cars were once a ticket to freedom, we are now hostages to our cars. Most of our cities and towns are such that we need a car to survive. We need a car to get food, to access decent housing, to find employment, to get to our workplaces and to entertain ourselves. If we don't have a car, or don't have access to one, we feel trapped, even helpless.

Most of us are all too familiar with that feeling. For me, one teenage incident in particular stands out. As a reckless sixteen-year-old, I drove my old Chevy Impala to the high school parking lot one night and did donuts until the engine died. I had to get it jumped by my parents, who were so upset, they took away my keys for a week. At the time, it felt like a social death sentence. How could I possibly have a life if I didn't have my car?

Perhaps you can remember a time in your life when you didn't have a car. Did your car break down and you couldn't

## Futurama

The classic example of the allure of the car age is General Motors' Futurama exhibit at the 1939 World's Fair. The exhibit portrayed a future world of people speeding along on free-flowing highways in cars, unencumbered by the old, cluttered city. In recent years, it even inspired an animated television series. There's a great video on the history of Futurama exhibit on youtube: http://www.youtube.com/watch?v=-JFgpxYaeJQ.

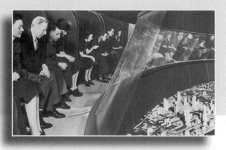

*People were enamored of Futurama.*

afford to fix it right away? Or was it in the shop for a few days? Did you injure yourself in a way that prevented you from driving? Did you lose a job and just couldn't afford a car?

It's for all these reasons and more that I love walking and choose to live in a walkable neighborhood. Because I am not dependent on my car, I have more freedom of movement than the average American. I'm never trapped at my house or apartment because of a car problem. If my car breaks down, I can still walk, ride a bike or take public transportation very easily to everywhere I need to go. I might even decide not to fix the car for a while, since I rarely need it urgently. As someone who was raised in pretty typical suburban environments, it's hard to describe just how empowering this freedom feels.

A formative time for me in terms of beginning to change my views on car reliance was a summer spent in Paris. In 1993, as an undergraduate studying architecture, I went to Paris on a summer program. As students, we lived for most of the summer

## Checking in with Futurama

In 2013, driving is not as fun as in the early decades of the automobile. One consequence of our car culture is that since everyone drives, we have endless traffic. Roads tend to be big and ugly, not the romanticized roads of car commercials. The reality of our car-oriented lives is not quite what we predicted in 1939.

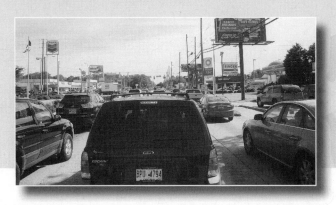

at the International University on the edge of the city center, just off the Boulevard Jourdan. Even without living in the heart of Paris, it was amazing to experience just how freeing it was to not *need* a car. Of course, we could rent a car if we wanted to (and we did, for one road trip), but we didn't need one for anything we did those six weeks. That forced experience of living a different way truly opened my eyes. Upon returning home, I honestly felt depressed at the lifestyle options presented to me.

But, as I argue throughout these pages, our lifestyle options are broader than we may think. My experience was twenty years ago, and much has changed since then. American cities and towns have begun a rebirth, working to recapture some of the character they had a century ago, when people routinely traveled by foot. Some places are much further along in that process than others, but from coast to coast, this recognition

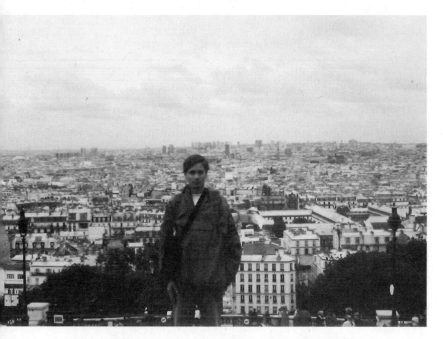

*Vive la France!*

of the importance of walkability has been a very encouraging phenomenon. Our communities increasingly allow us to walk to many destinations and experience a sense of the freedom I enjoyed in Paris. I found such a place in Savannah, Georgia. There are many others. And even if you don't live in a walkable place and are not about to pick up and move, there are still ways to incorporate more walking into your life — it just takes some creativity. Try it out for a time and experience the freedom that comes with more transportation choices.

I can actually (gasp!) eliminate my car if I so desire.

I grew up with cars, and for years I looked forward to the day when I'd own a car of my own. As a teenager in Marshall,

Missouri, there was nothing I wanted more than the freedom I thought a car would provide. I was raised on the idea of "cruising" as a fun activity, on my family's long road trips by car around the country, and on the notion that, on some level, our cars are an extension of who we are. Even when my friends and I were young and didn't have any money, we talked endlessly about what kind of beater we'd buy and how we would trick it out.

Feeling as if our cars defined us was not exclusive to young men. For many women of my generation and older, owning their own car was a way of establishing their place in the world, an expression of their independence from men. A good friend from high school, Renee Gentry, describes it this way: "Remember the Blue Bomber? My blue 1977 Chevy Impala with the 'upgraded' cassette deck? Nice. It was freedom. For me it was freedom in three significant ways: as a woman, as the youngest child and as a 'country kid.' I could listen to music *I* chose, not something picked by my older brother or sister. I had shared a room my whole life up to that point. This was the first thing I didn't have to share. I didn't have to rely on a 'date' to pick me up. I could literally 'go to town' and that meant I could get a job. It also meant, in my mind, that I could go to college someplace *else*."

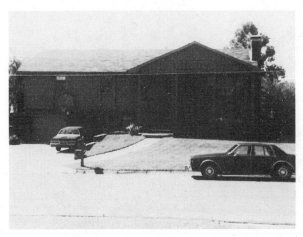

Freedom, as defined
by a teenager in
1987.

Given my history, the idea that I could potentially not have a car at all is, well, a little foreign and maybe even a little frightening. When I consider flat-out eliminating a car from my life, it feels a bit like I would be cutting off a limb. Even though I don't rely on it much anymore, there's a certain security in knowing it's there as an option. That's my context.

But as I age, and as I enjoy living a walkable life more and more, the idea of not having a car is becoming increasingly appealing in certain ways. I now run scenarios in my head of how

## Make Walking & Biking Easy Tip 2:
### *Have a Walking Station*

Keep a small cabinet near the front door to help with some of the daily routines of life. It's a great place to drop keys and wallets, keep an umbrella and more. Having all these items handy means you don't have them spread out all over the house, and it makes the act of coming and going much more brainless.

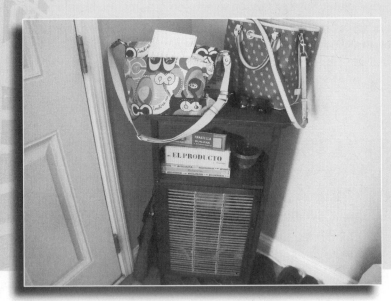

it would work, given my own travel patterns and my day-to-day life. How would I get to Target, for my occasional trip there? How about the beach or the movies? Would I take cabs to the airport?

The reality is that I have a choice. Should I want to sell my car and live without one, I can quite easily go on with my life and hardly notice a car's absence. I'm fortunate that for many of my daily needs, I can very easily walk or ride a bike. For longer or irregular trips, I could ride the bus or take cabs. I could even rent a car, should I want one for a day or more.

And there are still more possibilities for the car-less. The "sharing economy" is quickly expanding the options at my disposal. Car sharing, once available primarily in Europe and the largest cities in the United States, is quickly becoming an option in many more cities. Savannah doesn't have car sharing yet, but likely will within the next couple of years given how quickly it's catching on nationwide. Car sharing would allow me to have all the benefits of having a car when I need one without the hassles of owning one. And since I don't need a car very often, car sharing holds a good deal of appeal.

A great side benefit of living in a walkable place is that it's the kind of place where services like car sharing (and bike sharing, for that matter) make the most sense. Since members need

### JARGON ALERT: *Sharing Economy*

Maybe you've heard of Zipcar, Airbnb or bike sharing. These initiatives and more are termed the "sharing economy" because people are using modern communication technology to allow others to access the stuff they own. The websites and phone apps create trusted social networks and have a great side effect of people connecting more with each other in real life. It's a whole new approach to having access to the things we want or need in life.

## Sharing to Save

Bicycle Universe is a great website that includes information on the financial benefits of car and/or bike sharing: http://bicycleuniverse.info.

to get to a location where the shared vehicles are, which they generally do by walking, it helps to have those locations in walkable places. And since people who live in such places tend to own fewer cars and drive less, sharing vehicles better serves their needs than individual ownership. As our society continues to transition out of what I believe are the latter years of the car culture, it will be interesting to see how the "sharing economy" changes how we live.

Can the kid who grew up desperately wanting a car actually live without one? Increasingly, the answer is yes.

## I can take the bus, and no, it's not scary.

Let's be honest. For the majority of Americans, the bus is something we think only poor people use. They use it because they have to. And most likely, they do so because they can't afford a car. That's our impression. We feel badly for people riding the bus.

Like most stereotypes, there's a strong element of truth to this belief. Given how most of us have been raised (on the virtues of the car culture), the bus seems like a terrible alternative. I know that when I was a teenager, I couldn't wait to stop taking the bus to school and couldn't imagine choosing to use one as an adult.

Let's start with the negatives. Buses can in fact have seats that are a little too close to each other and be full of creepy-seeming people who don't smell great. The ride can bounce you around, and the driver may start and stop abruptly. The payment systems are often confusing. As for the routes, if you can quickly figure out where the buses are going and when by looking at signs on the street, then you're much more street-smart than most. So now that I've painted such a pretty picture, why would I suggest that taking the bus is a good thing?

Taking the bus is a little bit like eating brown rice or drinking fresh vegetable juice. We may not really like it at first, but it's good for us and we get used to it. Eventually, we might even enjoy it. One might say that taking the bus is an acquired taste. Every once in a while, I find myself taking the bus to downtown destinations in Savannah, either because of weather or my own laziness. I walk a few blocks to the stop and generally wait a few minutes for one to arrive. While the routes still seem bewildering at times, it's almost always a quick and easy trip that would otherwise take me thirty minutes or more to walk. Sometimes I even get a bonus of a good story to share with friends.

Bus systems can be confusing, and they can be a pain. But there are also a few pretty good things about the bus. They're hot in the winter and cold in the summer. They're an inexpensive way to go a long distance. Bus riders don't have to deal with parking, which is a notable benefit in some destinations. And because you're not behind the wheel, once you're on the bus you don't have to do a thing except sit back. When it's a longer trip, you can even read or watch movies. Oh by the way, you're also likely paying for the bus already with your tax dollars, so there's the financial element as well.

The same arguments can be made for trains, from streetcars to light rail to long-distance trains. As with buses, part of the joy of the train is removing the stress of driving and freeing up your time to do something else.

The good news is that smart people are working to make riding the bus a much better experience. Bus systems are adding services that are more reliable and upscale. If you have a smart-phone, you can pretty easily access bus schedules on it. Google Maps incorporates bus routes into its mapping, which is pretty cool. And many cities are redesigning their bus systems so that they are much more easily understood and go where people need them to go.

All this is well and good if getting to the bus is convenient for you, which typically means living in a walkable place. Since every

## Getting to Other Cities

It's also about buses or trains for long distances. I'm not in love with Amtrak or Greyhound, but those services do allow me to extend my walkable (i.e., non-car) reach. I can easily access the bus station or the train station without the need for a car (or at least with a short taxi ride), which allows me to travel to many different cities without ever getting behind the wheel.

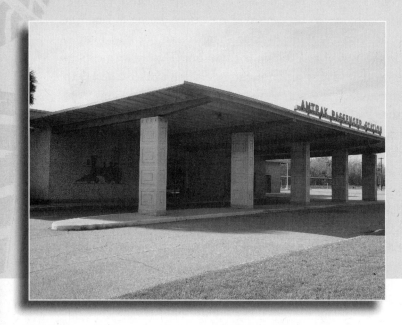

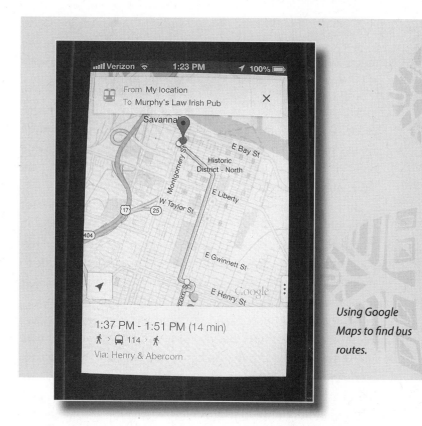

*Using Google
Maps to find bus
routes.*

bus trip presumably starts and ends with walking to the bus stop or having someone drop you off, getting to the bus is much more difficult if you live somewhere built for cars. The streets are filled with fast-moving traffic, and there may not even be any sidewalks. Walkable places have better bus service because they are walking places first — and because there are just more people to begin with.

So if you're one of the many who harbor negative views about riding the bus, know that you can change. I have — now I ride the bus on a regular basis. I doubt most of us will ever really love the bus. But hey, a little grilled chicken and vegetables over brown rice isn't such a bad idea once in a while.

## Walkable places are better for my kids.

OK, so I don't have kids. But if I did, I'd love for them to live in a walkable place and to be walkers like me. I've talked at length about how freedom of movement is a benefit to me, and I'll discuss some of the social and other benefits later. That same freedom is also available to children, especially those who are old enough to get out and about on their own.

Just think of some of the simple ways that life is better for both parents and kids in a walkable place. If there's a school in the neighborhood, they can walk to school (and home). They don't need me to drive them to the park, or to a store or to their friends' houses. They can even go to the store to get groceries for me, as kids did generations ago.

Those benefits may sound ridiculous or even terrifying to a lot of parents out there. Don't we live in a big, scary world with lots of crazy people? Why on earth would you want your kids out wandering around unsupervised? It is unfortunate that we live in a time and in places where horrible things can happen, and sometimes they happen to children. And it is absolutely true the world has its share of creepy and dangerous people.

## Child Abduction: Hype vs. Reality

*AOL News* published a fascinating piece in 2009 about the story behind child abduction statistics. Not only are missing children on the decline in general, but only a tiny percentage of missing children are actually abducted by strangers. It turns out half are runaways, and most of the rest are abducted by family members.

*(Source: "Child Abductions: The Hype vs. the Reality," AOL News. http://www.aolnews.com/2009/11/13/child-abductions-the-hype-vs-the-reality/.)*

But if we step back and review actual data, the statistics indicate that the things we most fear are very rare, and, in fact, the instances of violence against children have been growing less and less common. It often doesn't seem that way because our news media is so pervasive. When crime happens anywhere, it's very quickly national news. The attention and hype given to every singular event plays to our deepest irrational fears and has us asking, "Can that happen here?"

Look, life can be scary at times. But if we succumb to our fears, we give up the joys and pleasures of life, and that translates to our kids as well. Where once we allowed kids to play outside with abandon, we now confine them to only certain approved activities and locations. Where once it was common to walk to school, it's now the norm to be driven to school. When I was in elementary school, for example, after-school time often included walking along with friends to someone's house and impromptu games or goofing around. Today, parents who allow their kids that kind of freedom are almost considered neglectful. Instead, we somehow think it's safer and better to pile kids in the car, chauffeur them around and get them quickly to the house and backyard, or the supervised sports activity.

When considering safety, there are additional factors to keep in mind when thinking about turning kids, or even adults, loose.

### JARGON ALERT: *Eyes on the Street*

Renowned author and activist Jane Jacobs popularized the term "eyes on the street." Jacobs was a citizen activist and city lover, and she fought against the planning paradigm of the 1960s that was destroying pedestrian life in favor of easy driving. She wrote persuasively on how the concentration of people in cities makes those places safer because more people are watching.

Walkable places tend to have qualities that law enforcement personnel actually prefer because those places are safer. What are those qualities? For starters, more people on the street tend to mean more witnesses, which is generally a deterrent to crime. And in places that are best for walking, the houses typically open up to the front, often with attractive porches and stoops. The people who sit on those porches become "eyes on the street," helping to reinforce the safety of a place.

In fact, what we often don't think about is that the most dangerous places for kids are those places where they spend a lot of time: in cars. More children die from injuries in car accidents than anything else. That's true for every age group except those under a year old. Car accidents kill more kids than disease, birth defects or homicide. And millions more children are injured in car accidents. The National Library of Medicine and National Institutes of Health have documented the top causes of death for children and adolescents at this website: http://www.nlm.nih.gov/medlineplus/ency/article/001915.htm.

It doesn't have to be this way.

Beyond the safety issue, having more mobility and independence is better for child development. Kids need to be able to expand their world in ways beyond the video games in the basement. Sociability is incredibly important for children to learn at a young age, and the only good way to learn it is by meeting a

## Policing, Crime and Walkability

Police departments across the country ascribe to something called *CPTED — Crime Prevention Through Environmental Design*. Essentially, it's a set of policies that reinforces the safety benefits of walkable, active places. A good primer can be found on Wikipedia at: http://en.wikipedia.org/wiki/Crime_prevention_through_environmental_design.

wide variety of people in the course of daily life. That's far easier for kids to do when they can get out and walk around, or ride a bike around safely, than if they're stuck on a cul-de-sac waiting for their parents to take them somewhere.

Mobility is important for all of us, not just those of us who have the choice of driving. Kids want to explore their world. We need to make it easier for them to do so.

One of my favorite parts of the newspaper when I was younger was a small weekly article in which people wrote about their experiences as children growing up in Kansas City in the decades from the 1910s through the 1960s. Part of what struck me was how fondly and readily they talked about taking the streetcars with their friends, without adult supervision. They would walk alone or with friends to the neighborhood store or ride a bike to the park. Kids a century ago had much more freedom than kids today. The National Center for Safe Routes to School reported on this in its November, 2011 study, "How Children Get to School." The study found that even as recently as 1969, forty-eight percent of all kids walked to school. Now only thirteen percent do.

We all have fears about our world. It's unfortunate that this fear has caused us to give up so much. Childhood adventures are precious, and they are necessary for developing a sense of independence and engagement with the world. Not only does childhood independence help with sociability, it also builds confidence and self-esteem. As we rediscover walking, I hope we can find a way to make it a kids' paradise as well.

If I want to extend my reach, it's easy to hop on a bike to get farther.

When I was a kid in Albert Lea, Minnesota, the bike was my primary means of getting around — once I was too big for a Big

Wheel, that is. I loved getting on my bike and riding to friends' houses, parks, lakes and other destinations. I was fortunate that I lived in a small town where biking was easy and safe, in no small part because there was a large network of bike trails and bike routes.

As an adult, I still enjoy biking. My bike now is considerably more expensive and fancy, but it serves the same purpose — it further enhances and facilitates my experience of getting

### Make Walking & Biking Easy Tip 3:
*Keep the Bike Somewhere Accessible*

The easier it is to grab your bike and go, the more likely you are to use it. Consider keeping the bike on a porch (locked up of course), in a backyard that has gate access, or in a closet near the front door. If you're in a multi-story building, you must find a place to store it on the ground floor near the door. One company has devised a clever solution called the "bike shelf" that helps make storing a bike inside more fashionable: http://www.remodelista.com/products/the-bike-shelf.

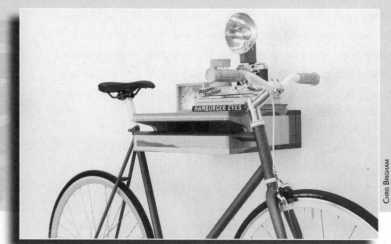

Chris Brigham

## Cyclist's Paradise

Denmark has become a cyclist's paradise, renowned for how it has made biking accessible for virtually everyone. In Copenhagen, fifty-eight percent of the population uses a bike daily. Slate.com published a great article in 2012 detailing what's been done there: "Can America Embrace Biking the Way Denmark Has?" (access it at http://www.slate.com/articles/health_and_science/the_efficient_planet/2012/11/green_wave_can_the_u_s_embrace_biking_like_denmark_has.html).

around without a car. And, not to put too fine a point on it, but biking in a bike-friendly city is a lot more fun than driving.

I like to be as honest as I can — both with myself and others — about what it's really like to be less car-dependent. I do love to walk, and I can often walk to quite a few daily destinations. But let's face it — some places are far away, some days I just don't feel like it, and some days the weather isn't great. On occasion, I'll hop in my car to take care of what I need to. But at other times, the bike is great for getting somewhere a lot faster than I can on foot.

The places that I most often go on a daily basis are generally within about a mile of where I live. With a bike, it's very easy to stretch that to two, three or even five miles.

For years, we've neglected the potential of biking as a viable transportation method. While many European nations have taken great strides in making biking comfortable and a viable option for everyone, we've tended to accommodate only the most avid cyclists. You've seen them, right? Wearing brightly colored, tight-fitting (sometimes too tight) clothes, the true warriors on bikes will ride anywhere, in any kind of condition. They spend a lot of money and time on the bike, doing routine rides of fifty or one hundred miles.

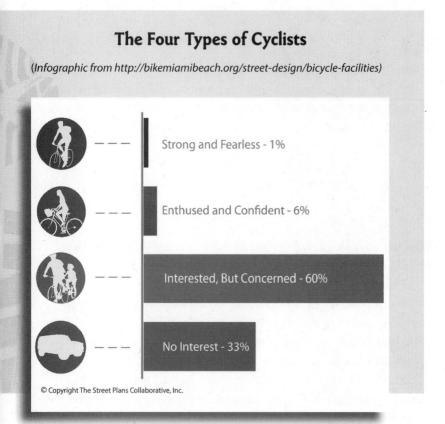

The Four Types of Cyclists

*(Infographic from http://bikemiamibeach.org/street-design/bicycle-facilities)*

Strong and Fearless - 1%

Enthused and Confident - 6%

Interested, But Concerned - 60%

No Interest - 33%

Good for them. But that's not me.

And, frankly, bike warriors are only a very small percentage of the US population. Cycling experts I work with tell me only one to three percent of the public are avid cyclists. Most of us fall into the large category of "interested, but concerned." By that, they mean we are interested in the idea of biking more, but concerned about safety, cost, road conditions, locking the bike, etc.

The good news is that our cities and towns are getting better at addressing our concerns. Programs such as bike sharing are on the rise, which make it easy to ride even if you don't own a bike.

## City Biking Version 2.0

Two of the best improvements in recent years for cycling are bike sharing and cycle tracks. The former is a very easy system to use a bike you don't own, and the latter is a next-generation bike lane that is protected from cars.

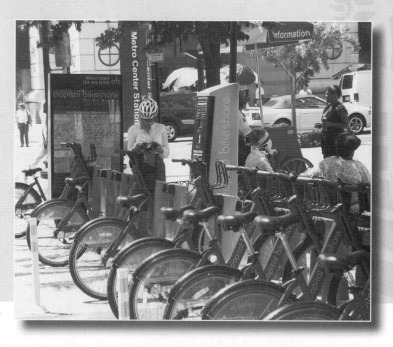

Physical improvements like cycle tracks and off-street bike paths are going well beyond the sad-looking bike lanes that were the first-generation efforts to accommodate cyclists. More cities are adding bike parking areas and bike racks that make it harder to steal a bike.

Like many of the subjects addressed in this book, the world of biking is looking brighter. For me, biking is just one more way to explore my world, get to where I need to go, and save a few bucks in the process. I'd also mention the exercise benefits, but that's for a later chapter. One of the best parts is that all those years of riding a bike as a kid have not gone to waste. It really is easy to pick it up again and remember the fun you had from long-gone days.

## I have a lot of different options for my routes.

"Variety's the very spice of life, that gives it all its flavour," wrote the poet William Cowper. And Robert Frost wrote, "Two roads diverged in a wood, and I — I took the one less traveled by. And that has made all the difference."

Both of these men speak to something deep within us as human beings. We like to have options. Options are good. Choices are good. Having choices in all matters of life feeds our senses of self and freedom.

I often hear people talk about making a place more walkable, and they start by complaining of a lack of sidewalks. That's a good place to begin, but it doesn't rate nearly as important as two other factors that I am able to benefit from every day in my neighborhood. One is the availability of destinations worth walking to. And the second is a wide variety of routes that I can take to get there.

The first item is obvious. If we don't have interesting places to walk to, our desire to walk is dramatically reduced. We may enjoy the recreational nature of getting out and going for a walk, which there's nothing wrong with, but it's not the kind of walking I'm writing about it in this book. What I'm describing is walking to the kinds of daily destinations that fill up our life: a school, a store, a coffee shop, a park, a restaurant, an office, etc.

The second item, however, is something that is all-too-often overlooked. As Mr. Cowper and Mr. Frost described, we crave variety. If I have only one walking route I can take to get to my destinations, walking quickly begins to feel less interesting and

*Which place has more options for walking, biking and driving?*

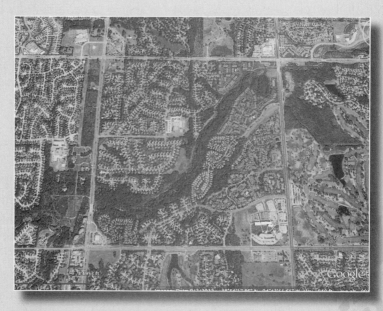

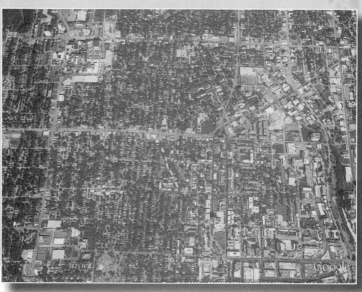

more like a chore. If I have a variety of paths I can take, I am much more interested in getting out and going. Depending on the weather, my mood, what I'm aiming to do, or who I might be walking with, I can select a path that fits the moment.

In urban planning terms, we call this variety a *network* of streets or paths. The network is more than a sum of its individual parts. A simple grid of streets, for example, can exponentially increase my options compared with a street network that provides only a couple of ways around.

Since most of our communities built before the 1940s were places where people walked daily, they are designed in this fashion. Following World War II and the adoption of the car culture, we radically changed our cities and towns so that they suited fast-moving cars. Planners and traffic engineers came together to create a new system of streets, giving them names such as *collectors, arterials,* and the now-ubiquitous *cul-de-sac.* Instead of a connected network, the new system was conceived to work like modern sewage systems, where cars were collected from endpoints and distributed to larger and larger pipes as they moved along. This approach fit the technocratic spirit of the era, as we believed rational, industrial mindsets could solve all manner of problems with city life. Cars became easier to count, and highly sophisticated traffic management systems were put in place. Alternate routes were limited on purpose, since traffic had to be contained to where it would cause the least negative impacts. Walking and biking were considered solely as recreational. We created a world based around the mobility the car provided, but in a twist of fate gave ourselves far fewer options for total mobility.

Another bit of simple truth: It's very difficult for planners to modify our car-oriented places so that they are interesting and useful to walk around. The streets are often so long that they are boring, and the destinations are spread so far and wide that walking is very inconvenient. Because of the design of the arterial-collector system, very few alternate paths exist. And, some of those other paths are not pleasant to walk along because of the traffic. It's simply a different system, with a different set of transportation priorities. This is not to say it's impossible to make changes or improvements in this environment, but it's certainly very difficult.

In our older places, however, the bones of good networks still exist. The cities are built with simple grids of streets, the blocks tend to be shorter, and the destinations are closer together. In my particular case in Savannah, I have a virtually endless number of choices for which way to walk on any given day. That set of options not only adds interest to my errands, but it also allows me to see more of my neighborhood and more of my city as a result. I am never bored.

The funny coincidence of living in a place that is more connected and has a finer network of streets is that it is not only better for walking — it also has benefits for driving. When I choose to drive, my routes are more direct. I don't have to drive a long way out of my way to go a short distance, which is very common in our newly built areas. And since I have a great number of streets to choose from when driving, I can easily avoid any congestion or emergency by just sliding over to the next street. Some people might call that a win-win.

In any case, there's no question that having variety and choices takes a simple walking experience and makes it a daily pleasure.

## If streets are closed for public events, it doesn't disrupt my life.

I'm not only a walker, I'm also a runner. I'm not hard-core, mind you. I'll run a few times a week, and do a 5K, 10K and even a half-marathon occasionally. Some of my real running friends would say that's pretty light, but I prefer to think that they're a little bit nuts.

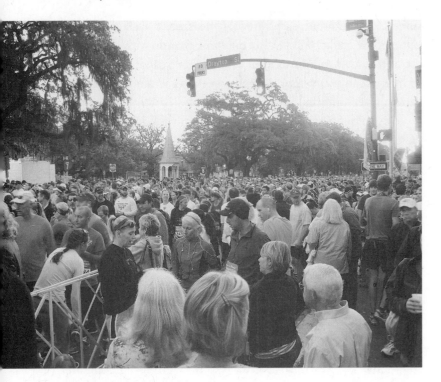

*Runners take over in Savannah.*

A lot of people get annoyed with how often the streets of their city are closed down because of races or special events. As running has increased in popularity, it's common in most cities to have an event of some kind almost every weekend when the weather is nice.

Races are hardly the only events that force temporary street closings. Street parties, parades, festivals, open street days, or even visits by dignitaries can all cause significant disruptions to the flow of cars through a city. Commuters hate having to deal with these situations, as there's nothing worse than being stuck in traffic with no options.

Although I've already established the virtues of having a network of paths to take in the previous section, allow me to add one additional benefit of having variety: I don't care when special events cause disruptions. In fact, it's even one better than that. As a walker, when streets are closed for events, I actually get to enjoy them. They don't affect my life in a negative way.

## Takin' It to the Streets

Initiated in Bogota, Colombia, *Ciclovia* is a day when a street or several streets are closed to traffic so that people can walk, bike or just hang out in the street. Many cities use Sunday as the day, since it's a slower day for traffic anyway. Since its start a few years ago, the idea has spread around the world, spawning the "open streets movement" in the United States. Look for one in your town.

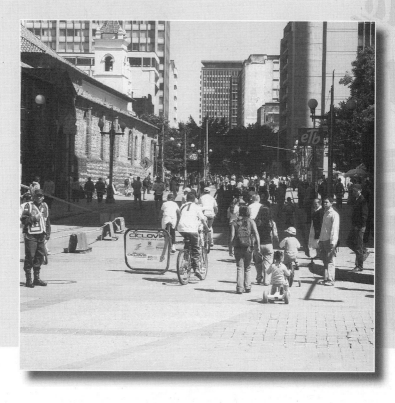

Now that I'm immersed in a culture of walking and biking regularly, when I hear people complain about big public events, I feel sorry for them. I feel bad that they feel so rushed in their days that they can't stop and enjoy the sights and sounds of people gathering together for fun. I feel sorry that they are more worried about getting to a store across town than about enjoying the moment. It's these kinds of spontaneous gatherings of people that we revel in when we're on vacation. And yet, when we return to our daily lives, we too often curse them.

I've even heard people say things to the effect of, "There's going to be a festival every damn weekend before long." Which makes me stop and wonder — would that really be such a bad thing?

## Snow days are great days.

I don't live in a snowy climate anymore, but one thing I surely miss is snow days. I miss those absolutely wonderful days when the sky dumps enough snow that it disrupts everyone's life.

Why do I so love snow days? Because in a walkable place, snow days are great days. I can get outside, walk around, and

## Talk about the Weather

Think it's too cold or too hot or too rainy to walk frequently where you live? Maybe it's time to do some rethinking. Copenhagen, Denmark, has a climate similar to Toronto's, yet it has a nearly unmatched walking and biking culture. Paris and London, known worldwide as "walking cities," have climates much like Seattle. Cartagena, Colombia, a unique and incredibly walkable city, is hotter and more humid on average than any city in the United States.

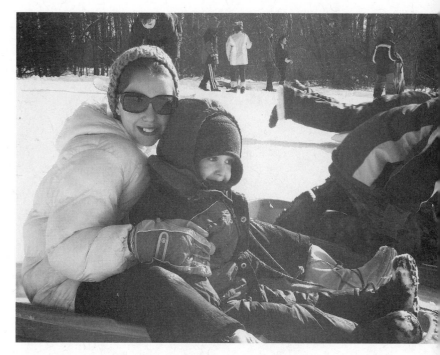

*Snow days are meant for kids.*

just enjoy the beauty and fun of it. I can still walk to stores if I need to, and I'm not consumed with what conditions the roads are in.

And of course, for kids, a snow day is nothing but fun. Having a nearby park with a hill for sledding is as fun as it gets.

A snow day is also one of those rare moments when you really notice just how much of the noise of life comes from vehicles. When the snow comes, the whole city gets eerily quiet, even in the midst of a major metropolis. Sounds that usually go unnoticed become audible. And the sounds we are more used to hearing (from traffic, trucks and sirens) are mostly absent.

I sure don't miss the cold weather, but I do miss those wonderful days where the snow makes it all shut down, and life gets a lot simpler.

## Why They Walk

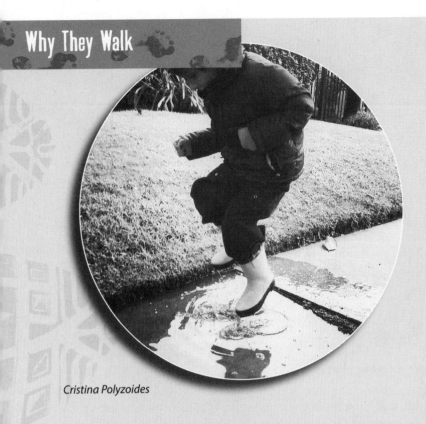

Cristina Polyzoides

*There is an old New Wave song that claims, "Nobody walks in LA" In my experience as a lifelong resident of the city, this isn't true.*

*For my family, walking in LA offers a variety of experiences. One is that the myth of our weather being the same all year has been dispelled. My husband and I have a five-year-old son, and our walking rituals change with the seasons. In fall, we collect leaves from our neighbors' trees for our nature table. Winter means rain boots and splashing in puddles. Spring marks the return of slow walks home from the Farmer's Market, and summer guarantees a stroll after dinner before bath, books and bedtime. The variety of the flora in this part of the world is breathtaking, and we enjoy the theatrics of nature, as well.*

*Another is seeing, firsthand, variety in the socioeconomics of our city. From time to time, we pass homeless people on the street, most in compromised mental conditions. We live a few blocks away from a large hospital complex, and it is very common to see men and women in scrubs walking to and from the campus. Then there are everyday folk at bus stops, pushing their children in strollers, walking home from the supermarket, engaged in their daily rituals. They are black, Latino, Russian Armenian, white, Pacific Islander, Asian, and in some cases, a mix of these ethnicities. Our son regularly sees signs in windows, billboards and other marketing material in languages other than English, and he is beginning to recognize that they are languages other than his primary one.*

*We believe that exposure to life as it is in our neighborhood, without the filter of a vehicle, is as valuable an element of our son's development into a well-rounded human being as is sending him to the school we have chosen for him. Life in all its forms on the natural to cultural continuum is shaping his mind and heart, not to mention those of his parents. We are fortunate to live where we do.*

— Cristina Polyzoides
Los Angeles, CA

# 2ⁿᵈ Interlude — *Sashaying to optional places*

Of course, not every destination is necessary: many are just for entertainment. Here's a few such places that I find myself walking to frequently.

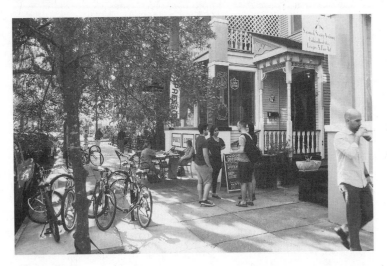

*Coffee shop.*

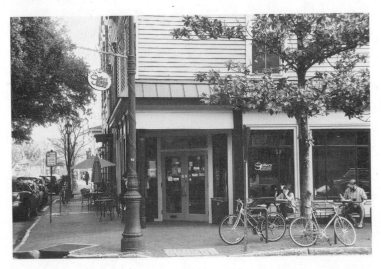

*Another coffee shop.*

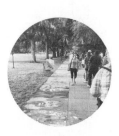 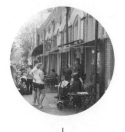 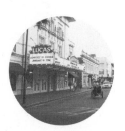

Yes, another coffee shop

Theater

Art Museum

Beer, Food & Trivia

Best burgers around

Pub

One of my favorite treats

My friend Stu's house

My friend Danah's stoop

Forsyth Park (where there's always something going on)

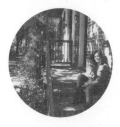 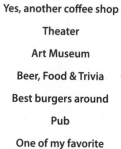 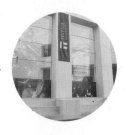

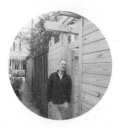 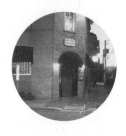

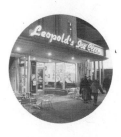 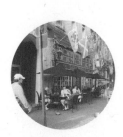 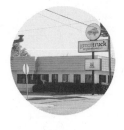

From the movie *LA Story*
  **Sara:** *Why don't we walk?*
  **Harris:** *Walk? Ha ha ha! A walk in LA!*

**4**

# Why I Walk: *Health*

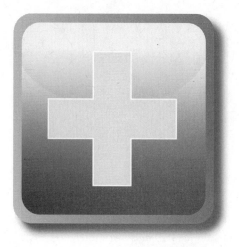

*Take a walk outside — it will serve you far more than
pacing around in your mind.*

— Rasheed Ogunlaru

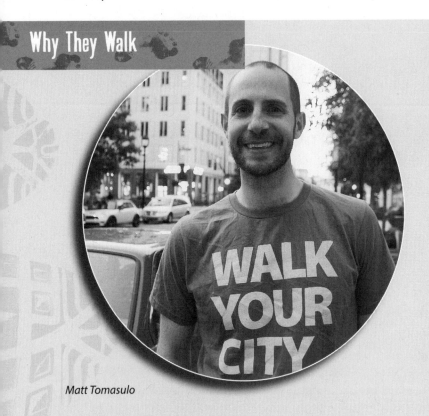

Matt Tomasulo

It is rather fitting that Kevin invited me to contribute to this book at this particular moment, for two reasons. Exactly one month ago, I decided to launch a new company called Walk Your City. Walk Your City is the result of a guerrilla wayfinding project I deployed one year ago in downtown Raleigh, NC, to bring awareness to the walkability in downtown. Secondly, I just made a decision to change my lifestyle: I moved into an apartment in the heart of downtown Raleigh, two blocks from the Capitol Building. Deciding to move was difficult and took a lot of thought because the cost of living in downtown Raleigh is twenty to thirty percent more than similar housing only a couple miles away.

I have lived in Raleigh for five years with a short stint in Carrboro, NC, while I was at UNC for two semesters. Since I moved to Raleigh,

I have made sure to live within a mile or two of school or work so that I can walk or bike. Raleigh is not a "walkers' paradise" and was just crowned with "most daily commute miles traveled," registering 37.5 miles per citizen, per day. Even in a city that averages over an hour of time in the car a day, I have managed to keep my commutes to ten minutes or less, on bike or foot. For 1.5 years during those 5 years, I did not have a car in Raleigh, one of the most autocentric cities in the country.

The choice to walk has stuck with me ever since I lived in Copenhagen, Denmark, for six months. My walks allow me to know my neighbors and neighborhood better. By choosing to walk, I will by default be closer to more people. For me, human interaction is very important. I have a greater sense of community and safety in the neighborhoods I have lived in over the past five years primarily because these walkable areas have more people living closer together, resulting in more human interaction.

Walking (and biking) is very important to me and my independence. Walking rejuvenates me. Walking is my own personal time, my chance to take that deep breath and not think about my inbox or Twitter feed. Walking brings clarity to my daily routine. My morning walk is my preparation for the day, my focus. Driving is not bad by any means, but it is certainly not relaxing, especially in Raleigh. When I drive, my anxiety increases, even on a short trip to the store a couple miles away.

I walk because the city is beautiful. I walk as my commute, but I also walk to meetings, dinner, to meet friends and during meetings. My office is in a quaint streetcar suburb of Raleigh that is across the street from a decommissioned four-hundred-acre mental hospital, and it just happens to have the best view of downtown.

My office is only two months old, but I have already gone on five different walking meetings through the Dorothea Dix campus. The loop we take is about forty-five minutes, which sets a great pace to our conversation and allows for exploration and exercise while *stimulating the conversation. Walking side by side during a business meeting completely changes the dynamic and has directly proven to help build better relationships with those folks who were open to taking a walk than were not.*

— Matt Tomasulo
Raleigh, NC

This may be the most obvious statement in the book and one that you don't need me to tell you, but bear with me: walking is good for you. Using your body to get around is much better for you than sitting in a vehicle. Our bodies were designed for being upright and getting around on our own two feet, not for sitting in one position for extended periods of time. It's no coincidence that the epidemic of obesity in the United States came about as we shifted into a more sedentary lifestyle with cars as the centerpiece.

## I am healthier.

Walking is so basic, and it's such an unconscious function that most of us don't stop to think about it, much less realize the potential impact of making a conscious decision to walk more. For example, I walk, on average, about two miles per day (when I account for all of my errands and pleasure walking). Some days it might only be a mile, while on others I cover much more ground, but I've tracked it, and that average basically holds. (If you want to measure your own walking, you can find some simple devices and phone apps, or websites like Google Pedometer.)

Those two miles per day work out to about 250 calories per day that I burn instead of, as Mr. Potter from *It's a Wonderful Life* says, "sitting on my brains." Those 250 calories are not a

## Sit on It

The conversation about how much time we spend sitting instead of upright is ramping up in the health and fitness community. Researchers are now studying how all of our sedentary activity is affecting our bodies and health. People are even promoting "stand up" desks at office places, as one remedy. You can look up a 2011 story on this topic, "Sitting all day" on www.npr.org (http://www.npr.org/2011/04/25/135575490/sitting-all-day-worse-for-you-than-you-might-think).

life changer, but as anyone who cares about fitness knows, every little bit helps. That amount alone accounts for a small meal or a couple of beers. As a frequent consumer of a couple of beers, I appreciate what walking does for my waistline.

And speaking of food, I regularly enjoy one important habit related to walking, which is taking a walk after eating. I enjoy good food of all kinds, and I occasionally overdo it at the dinner table, whether eating out or at home. But one thing that always eases the post-meal bloat is getting out and walking, even for just five or ten minutes. In my case, since I have a nice variety of restaurants and cafes to walk to regularly, I am able to walk off that meal on the way home. The post-dinner walk not only feels good physically, but helps my state of mind — making me feel just a little less guilty about having that last bit of...whatever.

Beyond the daily impact that comes from calories burned, there's also the cumulative effect of all that physical activity that is much harder to quantify directly. Using our bodies more regularly helps our overall fitness, including our cardiovascular health, our immune system, and the bones, joints and muscles in our bodies; exercise also has spin-off emotional and mental health benefits. Regular exercise of any kind is good, but the low-impact nature of walking has been shown to be better than many

## *How Many Calories Are in That?*

Take note: a two-mile walk takes care of the calories in all of the following:

- Beer, regular, 12 oz: 153 calories
- Red wine, 5 oz: 123 calories
- Slice of pepperoni pizza: 298 calories
- Scoop of vanilla ice cream: 145 calories
- Ground beef patty, 4 oz: 193 calories

*(Source: http://recipes.howstuffworks.com/45-common-foods-and-the-number-of-calories-they-contain.htm)*

**Calories burned by thirty minutes of activity**

| Body weight | 125 lbs. | 155 lbs. | 185 lbs. |
|---|---|---|---|
| **Activity** | | | |
| Weight lifting | 90 | 112 | 133 |
| Running 10 min/mile | 300 | 372 | 444 |
| Walking | 120 | 149 | 178 |
| Biking | 240 | 298 | 355 |

*(Source: Harvard Heart Letter, Harvard Health Publications, July 2004)*

alternatives. Many different health organizations, including the American Heart Association, recognize this and recommend a minimum of thirty minutes of walking per day, five times per week. The following infographic shows the benefits.

Of course, it's very possible to walk regularly and still be overweight or unfit. Physical fitness is multi-variable and includes not only exercise but what and how much you eat, along with genetics and other factors. But despite the variables, regular physical activity is critical to good health.

Of course, walking for exercise doesn't only have to happen while "exercising." The goal is to increase our activity throughout the day. Upping our energy expenditure includes walking on escalators and moving walkways (not just standing still), and using stairs instead of the elevator when possible. All of these

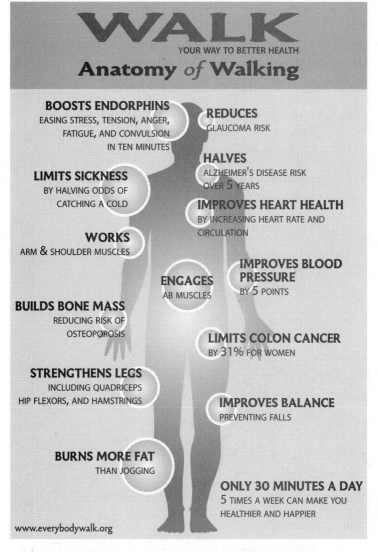

(Source: http://www.mindyourselfchicago.com/walk-your-way-to-better-health-infographic.)

strategies help build regular movement into our daily lives, help us get around and help foster good health.

Walking will not make you a healthy person in and of itself, but it's no coincidence that Americans walk far less on average than other countries and that we struggle more with obesity

## Is Walking Better Than Running When It Comes to Overall Health?

In the world of fitness, there's some debate about the virtues of walking for exercise versus running or other more vigorous activities. The American Heart Association gives this advice:

There are countless physical activities out there, but walking has the lowest dropout rate of them all! It's the simplest positive change you can make to effectively improve your heart health.

Research has shown that the benefits of walking and moderate physical activity for at least 30 minutes a day can help you:

- Reduce the risk of coronary heart disease
- Improve blood pressure and blood sugar levels
- Improve blood lipid profile
- Maintain body weight and lower the risk of obesity
- Enhance mental well-being
- Reduce the risk of osteoporosis
- Reduce the risk of breast and colon cancer
- Reduce the risk of non-insulin dependent (type 2) diabetes

Here's another article on the topic: http://www.straightdope.com/columns/read/2580/exercise-does-running-burn-more-calories-than-walking

## Endurance Walks, for Fun

It turns out, even Americans used to walk — a lot. Ten- and fifteen-mile walks were a routine occurrence in the days before the car, and not just because people had to. People did it because they liked it. It was a social experience as well as exercise. Today, many of us are hard pressed to walk even a half-mile without complaining.

(*Source: http://www.thesmartset.com/article/article12211201.aspx.*)

than anyone else. A 2010 study even tallied up our walking deficit, and it was reported on in the *New York Times* (http://well.blogs.nytimes.com/2010/10/19/the-pedometer-test-americans-take-fewer-steps/.) It turns out we're only walking on average about half of what health experts suggest. I can't guarantee what walking more will do for your health, but there's no question in my own life that walking regularly has made me feel — and even look — healthier.

## I don't need to drive to exercise.

That sounds like a crazy statement, doesn't it? Why would I *need* to drive to exercise? But many Americans do. We think of exercise as something we do at the gym, and most of us have to drive there. The other option for most of us? If we get sick of the driving and the membership costs, we spend thousands of dollars on our own personal gym equipment, including treadmills and stationary bikes.

Is there anything more boring than riding on a stationary bike or running on a treadmill for a few miles?

I simply head out my door to exercise. Sure, if I want to lift weights, I need to either go to a gym or set myself up at home. But for walking — and for running and biking as well — I can do those very easily and safely in my own neighborhood. And it's not just that it's easy, it's also more enjoyable for me than being in a gym.

Whether walking, running or biking in my neighborhood, I have multiple paths I can take, as I discussed in Chapter 2. In addition, the streets are narrower than in a non-walkable neighborhood, and the cars are moving more slowly, so it's very safe for those of us moving around on two feet or two wheels. As an added bonus, my neighborhood has tree-lined streets and nearby parks that make these activities a true pleasure.

My frequent routine is to head to Forsyth Park and run the one-mile loop around the park, mixed in with some random running on neighborhood streets. Even if I keep to a similar path each day, it's never boring because the people along the way vary my experience each time. With a truly social place like a park in the neighborhood, I've got my own personal, live-action social network that's fascinating to observe and participate in.

Obviously, not every place has a setup like my neighborhood. And not even all quality walkable places have those kinds of amenities. But even without them, running or biking along any of the streets in a walkable place is preferable to doing these activities in a place that's not walkable.

It's instructive to compare Savannah's pedestrian-friendly nature with that of a pretty typical suburb, one in which it's not especially enjoyable to walk, run or bike (although I would still argue that it's better than driving everywhere). When I visit my parents in Lenexa, Kansas, I exercise by jogging in the

**FACTOID:**
American households spend an average of $130 per year on exercise equipment.

(*Source: http://www.livestrong.com/article/487016-the-average-money-spent-on-gym-equipment/*)

**Make Walking & Biking Easy Tip 4:**
*Get a Basket for Your Bike*

When riding a bike for utility instead of competition, it's highly advisable to get a basket for your bike. Fortunately, they come in a wide variety of shapes and sizes to suit your particular needs.

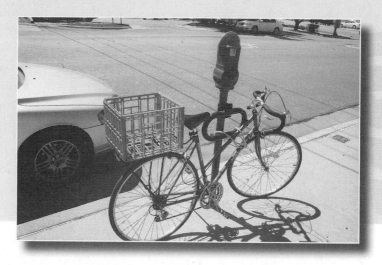

neighborhood. The challenge is that their neighborhood is like a lot of places we've built in this country over the past fifty or sixty years. The streets are set up primarily for cars to drive quickly, so it doesn't feel entirely safe to be out on foot. There are no parks or squares in easy walking distance that I might jog around (incidentally, this is something we can work on in all of our cities and towns). A bike/pedestrian path exists along one of the streets near my parents' house, but it's not shaded, and the street has very fast-moving traffic. Another unsatisfying feature of the path is that it's a singular experience, as it simply follows the roadway. The adjoining streets all have long blocks and frequent dead-ends, so the opportunities for different routes are limited. These factors combined make the experience of being

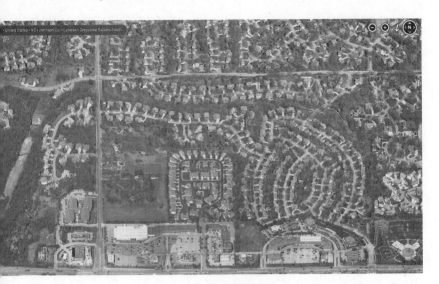

*Walking in suburbia is neither easy nor enjoyable.*

out and about less enjoyable than in my neighborhood. And if it's less enjoyable, I'm less motivated to get out and do it.

Exercise is something most of us are rarely very eager to do. At the same time, we all know the important health benefits of exercise. It's so important that we go to great lengths to make sure we squeeze it into our day. Living in a place that subtly encourages you to get out and about is one more benefit of a pedestrian-friendly place. Many days we simply don't have the willpower to make a big effort. On those days, it's great to be in a place where twenty minutes working out is just that, not twenty minutes plus another thirty minutes in traffic.

## Driving less is better for my blood pressure.

I'm one of those drivers you hate. When I'm behind the wheel, I tend to shift personalities and become an aggressive driver who speeds far too often. My driving record reflects this tendency, although I'm amazed I haven't been busted more often for speeding.

Even worse, I tend to get road rage. George Carlin once famously said, "When you're driving, everyone else is either an idiot or a maniac." I completely identify. Nothing gets me more worked up than what I see as the stupid things other drivers

## Slowing Down

I can't write a book on walking versus driving without mentioning Hans Monderman. This unconventional engineer turned the field of road safety on its head with his groundbreaking theories and the successful projects that bear them out. His approach holds that actually removing stop signs, signals and other features creates situations in which drivers are forced to pay attention, and thus they do. I can relate. Experience has certainly shown me that just the presence of traffic signals feels like a free pass to accelerate. On the contrary, when confusion reigns, I slow down and pay close attention. Here's a video of a small town in England that recently utilized Monderman's techniques to great success: http://www. youtube.com/watch?v=-vzDDMzq7d0&feature=player_embedded

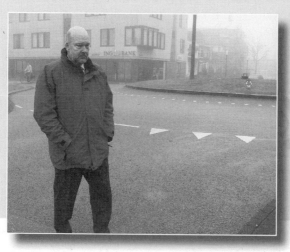

*Hans Monderman, Traffic Engineer and Innovator.*

routinely do behind the wheel. Whether it's that painfully slow right turn, the U-turner who doesn't quite make it the first time, or the slow driver in the fast lane — you name it. Do I do those things? Never...

It is interesting to me that when I walk, I tend to see people as people, and I'm quick to say hello or find something to smile about. Yet, put me behind the wheel of a car, and I end up cursing those same people as my blood pressure rises.

In my field, we often promote something called *Traffic Calming*, which is essentially a way to alter our streets so that drivers are forced to slow down. Anyone who drives has experienced this, although perhaps not consciously. I have a deeper understanding of the importance of this strategy than most people, because I'm the target driver. If the street design encourages me to go fast, such as with wide lanes and long views, I'll do so. If the street has more activity or seems the slightest bit confusing, I slow down.

Renowned Dutch traffic engineer Hans Monderman said of behavior like this, "If you treat people like idiots, they'll behave like idiots." He championed the design of streets and intersections that are intentionally confusing, so that people are forced to slow down and pay attention. Spoiler alert: It works.

## All Stressed Out

We know that stress affects us physically as well as mentally. It wreaks havoc on our entire body, from our emotional well-being to the functioning of our organs. But what do we do about it? Most physicians emphasize the importance of exercise and physical activity as a primary means of relieving stress. The light-impact nature of walking lends itself especially well to stress reduction. Here's a fact sheet on stress and how to manage it from the National Institute of Mental Health: http://www.nimh.nih.gov/health/publications/stress/fact-sheet-on-stress.shtml

I suppose to a certain extent it's natural that operating a heavy, rolling piece of machinery can affect our temperament. After all, we've got a lot of power at our disposal, both to take us long distances quickly and to potentially injure or kill another person. Driving *should* be a big deal, and it *should* give us heightened senses.

Walking, on the other hand, is calming. I do walk places in a hurry sometimes, and my mood at those times is slightly different. But even then, I'm far more forgiving of my fellow human beings, and I'm in no position to run them over with a ton of steel and plastic. When walking to a business lunch, I might quicken my step, but it's nothing compared to the stress of driving, parking and driving again in the same space of about an hour. Walking somewhere makes me noticeably more forgiving, patient and present in the moment. Life slows down, and for me that's a good thing.

I've never actually taken my blood pressure while driving (you're welcome) or while walking, but I can certainly feel the difference in the amount of tension in my body. How does your behavior change when behind the wheel?

## I stop and smell the roses, which is good for my mental health.

I don't often literally stop to smell the roses, though in spring I love to smell the jasmine. But walking does offer me the daily opportunity to enjoy the little interesting details of life. Since I'm not whizzing by at thirty or forty miles per hour, I find myself noticing beauty in far more places than is possible from behind the wheel of a car.

What are those little things? One day I might observe a detail on a porch or window that escaped my eye on my many previous walks. Another day I'll spot a new plant or flower that's blooming. Sometimes it's something as simple as water puddled up in the street that reflects light in just the right way. I often pause in Forsyth Park to watch the water reflecting the ever-changing light, or even the absence of it at night.

It's no mystery why places such as Paris and Rome evoke romantic ideals in our hearts. These places touch us because we

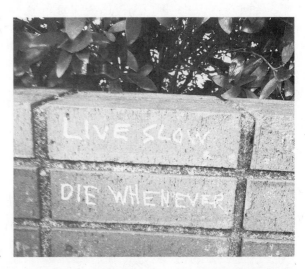

*Daily moments of joy.*

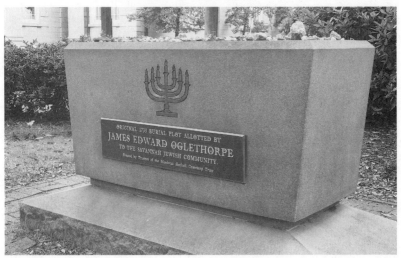

experience them slowly. The charm of the streets, the plazas and the architecture work wonders because we walk by them and notice. It's a world built for beauty and the experience of life at a slower pace.

That experience of beauty in my daily life helps to invigorate my mind and body. A walk down a beautiful street can change my mood and inspire me. Other people are obviously touched as well, since the most pleasing portions of my walks are full of fashion shoots and weddings, and I've even witnessed proposals in progress on more than one occasion. Beauty ultimately may be in the eye of the beholder, but we clearly have some deeply shared ideas about what makes places beautiful.

I should add that it's certainly possible to have a walkable place that is not beautiful. A neighborhood can have all the attributes I've discussed, such as important destinations, a network of streets and paths, and public spaces and yet be nondescript or even ugly. In fact, this scenario is not only possible, but also probable in a world of cheap and quickly built buildings.

When we allow people to create that ugliness, we deny something basic to our nature. Humans crave sensory experiences, and visual beauty is a key part of that. Places that technically work well, but are unattractive, will never touch us in the same way as places that are beautiful. To lack beauty in a place's buildings and landscape is like food without flavor. The food may provide necessary sustenance, but it won't provide the joy and pleasure we ultimately crave. And, I would argue, ugly places won't get us out and walking around as much, either.

## I'm greener, which makes me feel better.

I could devote this entire book to a discussion of the environmental benefits of walking and walkable places. In fact, numerous such books and reports have been written. Many of them are great, and I would never discourage anyone to dig deeply into the data.

But this is about a personal look at walking, not a societal one.

It should be obvious by now that walking more often, and driving less, means that I use less fossil fuel than I would otherwise. Since this is the case, I also contribute less to the problem of greenhouse gases. Simple enough: less fossil fuel has many benefits, as do fewer pollutants.

I like to do my part when I can to make the world a better place, and this is one important area that is in my control — it makes me feel good. My spending and lifestyle habits alone cannot significantly impact global energy issues, climate change

## Make Walking & Biking Easy Tip 5:
### *Keep Quarters Handy for the Bus or Get a Monthly Pass*

If you ride the bus frequently, the best thing to do is get a monthly pass. It makes riding so much simpler, and you don't have to ever worry about needing change. In a few years, I imagine we'll all have some version of "smart cards" that will make all transportation options easier, but for now we must have separate cards for all. If you don't ride the bus frequently, keep a bowl or container handy in your Walking

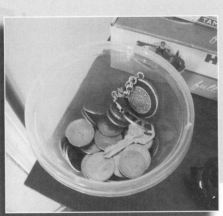

Station. Just dump spare quarters in the bowl when you have them, and grab and go when you think you might ride the bus.

## Walking Is Good for the Planet

The Internet is filled with references to the environmental benefits of walking. Walkinginfo.org is a good place to start. (http://www.pedbike info.org/data/factsheet_environmental.cfm)

or environmental pollution. One person's actions alone cannot save the world. But I can at least sleep better knowing that I'm making an effort.

I'm not advocating that we should all immediately give up our cars, start walking, wear Birkenstocks and eat only organic foods. But I do believe that as long as we live in a world of vast choices, everyone needs to consider what suits them best.

For me, personally, I care about what happens to the health of our planet. I care because the health of our planet affects my health and the health of others. If our water is polluted and I drink it, it will make me sick. The same goes for our air or our food supply. I don't like being sick, and I don't like my friends and family getting sick. I've coughed up unmentionable stuff from dirty air in China, and I don't want to live that way.

I also care about what is happening to our climate because of fossil fuel burning. I'm not a scientist, and even the best climatologists can't predict accurately what will happen as the planet continues to warm. But we do know that life sustains itself quite well under today's conditions, and I'd like for humanity to do its level best to not mess that up.

So another spin-off benefit for my mental health from walking is that I feel like I'm doing what I can in terms of the environment. I realize that it's not enough for just me to do this. But I can't control everyone else, nor would I want to if I could. We all make our choices. For me, it feels good to contribute.

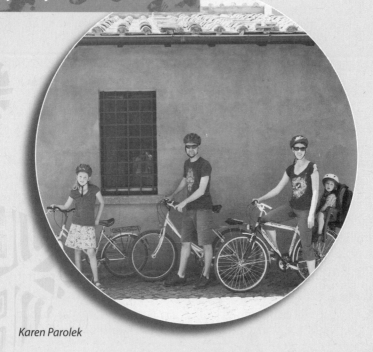

*Karen Parolek*

I was thirty-six years old before I owned my first pair of adult-sized rain boots. I don't remember if I had any as a kid, but it had never occurred to me to buy them as an adult. After buying my daughter a new pair each year for five years, I finally realized that I could buy my own pair, and I wouldn't even grow out of them in a year. Owning rain boots gives me the freedom to jump in puddles, which I do whenever I can. Better yet, I now own rain pants, a good rain jacket and rain fenders on my bike, so I can ride through puddles, spraying water everywhere. Enjoying a life of biking and walking keeps me young in so many ways.

On my bike ride home from work, I have found the perfect hill. It's a half-block long, perfect to go down full speed (without exceeding the speed limit) and still have room to glide to a stop before the next intersection. It's also been recently repaved, so the ride is smooth and glorious, like a perfect snow hill. A squeal often escapes my lips on the way down. I consider this hill my gateway between work and home, to release the work stress of the day.

I also ride my kids to and from school. My son, now three, rides his push-bike along the sidewalk, as I ride next to him in the street. He doesn't have pedals yet, which limits his speed and makes for easy stops along the way. When I'm in a hurry, this can be frustrating. My goal, though, is to use this time to live life closer to his preferred pace. I've learned to bring along my cup of tea, and every time he stops to look at a worm crossing the sidewalk or the water running under the bridge along the way, I take a sip of tea to remind myself to slow down and enjoy these moments.

My daughter, now ten, occasionally rides her bike home from school with her friends, sans adults. I have confidence in her ability to ride safely because I've made the same bike commute with her for six years. I've used that time to teach her how to ride safely and defensively, how to be considerate of others, and how the rules of the road work; essentially, how to be safe, responsible, courteous and independent. She has soaked these lessons up like a sponge because she was young enough to still listen to my input. If I had waited until she was fifteen to teach her the rules of the road, she might have cared less what I had to say about being courteous of others and taking her turn at the stop sign. By teaching her young, I have more trust that these things are part of who she is.

Riding my bike is a gift I give to myself. It's a way to remind myself of the parent and person I want to be. But mostly, it's just fun — splashing through puddles, squealing down hills, stopping to watch the worms with my son, and watching my daughter learn and grow. What could be better than that?

— Karen Parolek
Berkeley, CA

### 3rd Interlude — *Choosing not to saunter*

The neighborhood has a lot of other destinations that I could walk to, but for a variety of reasons, I choose not to.

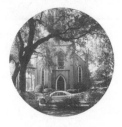

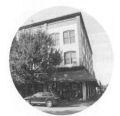

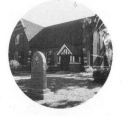

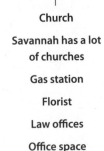

**Church**

**Savannah has a lot
of churches**

**Gas station**

**Florist**

**Law offices**

**Office space**

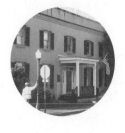

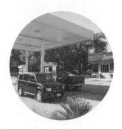

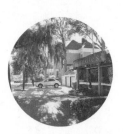

*I walk everywhere in the city. Any city. You see everything
you need to see for a lifetime. Every emotion.
Every condition. Every fashion. Every glory.*

— Maira Kalman

**5**

# Why I Walk: *Social*

*In Paris, with miserable weather, in thousands of outdoor drinking and eating places, the generations gather to talk and stare . . . which is what life is all about. Gathering and staring is one of the great pastimes in the countries of the world.*

— Ray Bradbury
*The Small-Town Plaza: What Life Is All About*

# Why They Walk

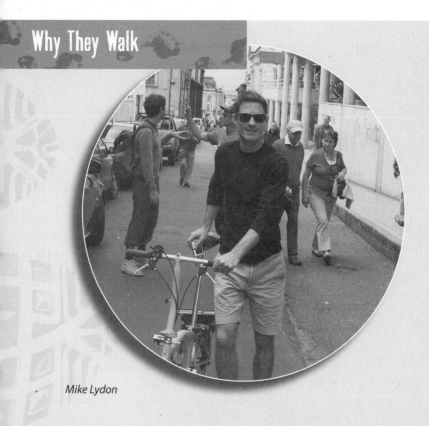

Mike Lydon

I grew up in midcoast Maine, where walkable villages dot a land-scape of pine trees and rocky peninsulas. When I was young, I took this beautiful balance of town and country for granted because I knew little else.

I now live in Brooklyn, New York. Life by foot is so convenient here that I often joke that great urbanism is for lazy people; the thought of driving somewhere for a slice of pizza, groceries, or a bottle of aspirin seems like an unnecessary, if not Herculean, effort.

Of course, New York is not a city of lazy people; it's full of go-getters like the man who sells newspapers at the mouth of the Clinton-Washington subway stop. We don't know one another's names, but we know each other. He watches me run to Prospect

Park and return forty-five minutes later. He knows when I have dirty laundry. And he knows when I've run out of milk. In turn, I know his favorite customers; it's written on their smiling faces like the morning headlines. I know that the woman who helps him on certain sunny days is his wife. And I know that the storage unit for his makeshift newspaper stand (two milk crates, a wooden chair and a particle-board plank) is the otherwise unused light well below my stoop.

Our unspoken relationship is just one of millions among dizzying permutations of New Yorkers crossing paths. But inherent to them all is the city's walkability — the very source of the newspaper seller's livelihood. As I walk down the stoop to the sidewalk and mount my bicycle bound for work, I look back at him and smile because I know that it's my livelihood too.

— Mike Lydon
Brooklyn, NY

No matter how much we strive for individual identity, we can't escape the fact that humans are social animals. We not only enjoy the social contact with others, we crave it. It's in our nature, and there's ample evidence that humans don't thrive in isolation. In small doses, sure, isolation can be refreshing. But too much of it does strange things to people. We're hard-wired to seek out other people in all sorts of situations and make connections, whether we're introverted or extroverted. You might even say the survival of the species depends on it.

## Walking is a fun social activity.

What I really enjoy about walking is that it fills that need for sociability, especially if you're in a place where there are lots of other people out walking. I think that's precisely why we tend to vacation in places where walking is the norm, because that sort of public socializing is something most Americans lack in their day-to-day lives. We get up, we drive to work, we drive to shopping, we drive to entertainment, and then we drive home. Sure, each of those individual activities may provide some social stimulation, but not the kind of relaxed, informal sociability I'm talking about.

What do I mean? The other day, Jamie and I were out walking, headed downtown to run a couple of errands and just enjoy a Sunday. On our walk downtown, we ran into our trivia buddy Roy walking in the park. At sixty-four, Roy is the social butterfly of Savannah (he still carries with him a desk-size written calendar of all of his activities), and he was checking out a group of young hippies in the park who have a new drum circle. The drum circle — that's a whole other story.

At any rate, running into Roy turned into a fifteen-minute conversation. We chatted about what was going on in the park, what we'd done over the weekend, and what was coming up during the week. Of course, we also talked a little about some mutual friends. I learned a new thing or two about Roy, and I'm sure he learned something about us as well. And, it was just plain fun — a happy interruption in the day.

The thing is, this type of random run-in happens all the time when you live in a walkable place. We've had days or nights out where we've bumped into several different friends from entirely different circles, all in just a few hours. And those encounters don't happen only inside a crowded bar or a noisy coffee shop. They happen outside, on the streets or in the squares, as we're going about our own fun. One of the primary characteristics of a great walkable place is how living outdoors in public becomes a much more frequent occurrence.

The kind of sociability I've described is not just fun (and interesting), but something most of us lack in our daily routine. Despite the romantic call to the wilderness, we humans need regular connection with each other as much as ever. There's simply no amount of Facebooking or social media that can replace it, no matter how sophisticated our technology becomes.

## I have more disposable time.

We think of cars as time-saving devices. If we want to get somewhere fast, the obvious solution is to get in the car and drive there. Cars can take us to faraway destinations relatively quickly if there's no traffic — as a result, we perceive car use as efficient time management, and even time gained.

What I've found is more often the opposite.

I've discovered that by walking and biking I spend *less* time getting to my destinations than when I drive. As a result, I now have more disposable time than I used to have.

I fully understand that what I'm describing won't be true for everyone, and it won't be true for every place. But here's how it works for me.

In my former home in Kansas City, I could walk to a few destinations that I went to regularly, but many others were so spread out that I had very little choice but to drive to most of them. For example, I had a nice selection of restaurants and coffee shops that were an easy walk. A few close friends lived within walking distance, and if the weather was nice, I could walk the twenty-five minutes or so to work. But my many business trips took me to offices around the city, most shopping wasn't convenient, and I often wanted to explore the food and drink options beyond my neighborhood. I could have taken the bus to some of those places, but the bus service in Kansas City was so bad that in most cases riding the bus took substantially longer than driving.

The situation I have now is quite different and, as I've mentioned, was a major factor in why I chose to move here. I have most of my daily and weekly destinations within a fairly easy walk. Ten to fifteen minutes from my front door gets me to many places I need to go, including all manner of food and drink options; local services like groceries, banks, barbers and doctors; as well as parks, recreation and even the very frequent festivals. The act of driving and looking for parking actually takes longer, in part because it's less direct and in part because parking is sometimes difficult to find. As a result, I spend far less time getting to destinations now, when I travel primarily by foot and by bicycle, than I used to when I drove pretty much everywhere — and much less than the average person spends.

**Average commuting times for select cities, each way**

| New York City/NJ/Long Island | 34 minutes |
|---|---|
| Washington, DC | 33 minutes |
| Chicago | 31 minutes |
| Atlanta | 30 minutes |
| Los Angeles | 29 minutes |

*(Source: US Census Bureau, American Community Survey, 2010)*

**Make Walking & Biking Easy Tip 6:**
*Use Google Maps for the Bus or Your Transit Company's Phone App*

Transit agencies have been slower to adopt smartphone technology than I would like, but most are finally getting on board. Google Maps is handy for searching for bus routes and times, though it is still somewhat imperfect. I expect this technology will only get more intuitive and customer-friendly over time.

In fact, the average American spends an hour and a half a day behind the wheel of a car. Just think for a moment how much time that is. Adding that up over the course of a year comes to about *three weeks* of time. The average commute in our country takes twenty-five minutes *each way*. And that's the average. In contrast, my average time behind the wheel is about two hours *per week*.

Of course, I trade some of that driving time for walking or biking time, but the difference is that the latter is time I generally enjoy. As mentioned earlier, walking is healthier, more relaxing, and just generally makes me feel good. Most importantly, I find that by living in this more compact way, I have additional time to do the things I enjoy. During those times when I am stuck in traffic, I find myself giving thanks that it is not part of my daily life.

Only by removing ourselves from the day-to-day grind of driving everywhere — which most Americans simply accept as part of living the good life — do we realize how poor that quality of time actually is. We've done our best to make sitting in the car as good as we can, with comfortable seats, premium audio systems and hands-free phone devices. But the reality is that it's a lousy way to spend ninety minutes a day.

Personally, I prefer to spend my time with friends and family or tinkering on my latest project, rather than behind the wheel.

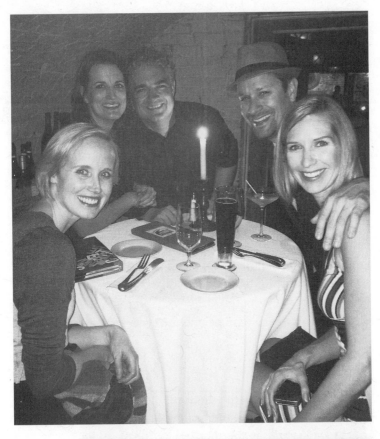

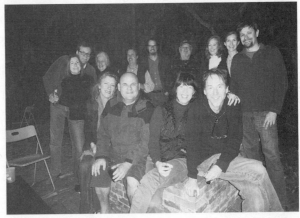

*Less time behind the wheel means more times like these.*

If I devote that extra time to being sociable, it helps strengthen my relationships. Other times, I want to dive into some personal hobby, or even relax and do nothing. Finding time for all of those activities is possible by choosing to drive less and live more.

## If I feel like socializing with my neighbors, it's easy.

I'm routinely reminded of the fact that not everyone is extroverted, as I tend to be. Many people get worn-out with too much human interaction and need to recharge in solitude. Still others are private people and generally limit their socializing. And all of us like being alone at times. Nothing is wrong with any of these personality traits.

But for those times when socializing is something I want to do, I've found it's far easier in a walkable place. When I wanted to meet my neighbors, or now, when I would like to know them better, the design of my neighborhood and its buildings allow that to happen more intuitively than in most suburbs. If I have friends who live within an easy walk, I'm much more inclined to visit them than if I had to drive. A ten-minute walk to say hi is a pleasant experience, whereas a ten-minute drive is long enough to keep me from making the trip.

A lot of people may question what I'm saying. After all, is it really that hard to get to know your neighbors, regardless of the setting? With a little effort, of course, it's not that hard to get to know people. But the design of a place does impact our behavior in both obvious and less-than-obvious ways.

The placement and details of our streets, buildings and landscapes can help or hinder human interaction. The smallest elements of design often alter our behavior in ways in which we are not aware. In community design, we see this routinely.

My brother is a psychologist, and we once hosted a discussion at his workplace about whether design can really impact the bonds of community. I was faced with a room full of skeptical PhDs, but, as a young architect, held my own in arguing the affirmative. My case boiled down to observed experience, though others have before and since completed detailed peer-reviewed studies. Consider it this way: think for a minute of a neighborhood where the buildings are fairly close to the street, the houses have front porches, and people regularly walk on the sidewalks. Compare that neighborhood to one typical of most of those we've built in this country in the last thirty or forty years. The streets are wider, there is probably a sidewalk on only one side of the street, garages dominate the houses, and in the absence of front porches, people generally hang out in their backyards. In which type of place do you think it's more likely for you to run into people casually, or feel encouraged to go knock on a neighbor's door?

I've lived in both kinds of places and can tell you there's a tangible difference in the social feel. This does not mean that I know all of my neighbors. But it's quite obvious that the opportunities to engage are easier and more frequent in my current neighborhood than in the more insular world of suburban-style streets.

Whether we speak or not, I certainly see my neighbors more frequently now than in my previous homes, and they no doubt see me as well. These kinds of public connections are significant because they reinforce good civic behavior, which I even notice in myself on occasion. Knowing that people will observe and register my actions, I am more likely to put trash where it's supposed to go, pick up the dog poop, clean up my porch, and generally behave more like a grown-up.

I'm not a sociologist, so I can't explain why these behaviors exist. But many good people have studied the ways in which our places impact our lives and have come to the same conclusions. We humans are subject to influence by a variety of design variables. And yes, some of those include the actual design of our neighborhoods.

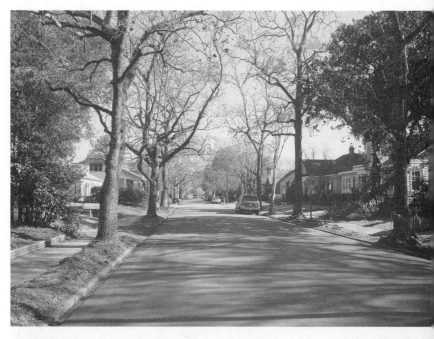

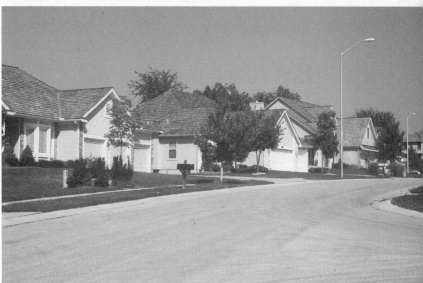

*Compare and Contrast: Which place looks more welcoming to you?*

## I learn more about my city.

Not all of the social benefits of walking will appeal to everyone. We all have different temperaments, interests and tastes.

I love to learn about the history of where I live. I can do that more easily as a walker than when I'm whizzing through the streets at thirty-five to forty-five miles per hour. When walking, the sights and sounds are up close and personal instead of flashes that disappear before I can identify them. I get to experience life at three miles per hour. At that pace, I get to see the details of my neighborhood and city. The signs that note the year of a building's construction or the monument to someone from

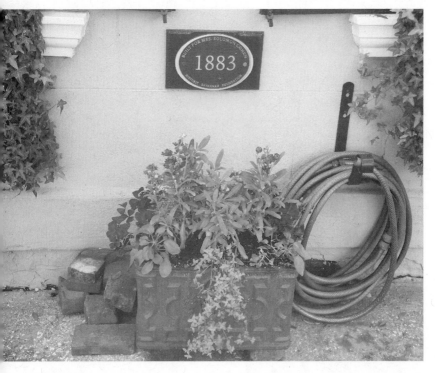

*Living history.*

**JARGON ALERT:** *The three-mile-per-hour city*

Danish architect Jan Gehl, who has contributed much to making Copenhagen pedestrian- and biker-friendly over the course of the last five decades, coined this term. Describing how to build at a human scale, he says:

> You put an emphasis on the people walking and bicycling and also on public life in general. That means you start with the people and end with all the other things. You have motor traffic and buildings as second priorities. If you don't start with the people side of the story, you can never add the people side after you have made cars happy and placed a number of buildings around a place. You have to start with the people. So that's one side of it. The other side is something which takes its point of departure in the human body and human senses. If you go to a place like Venice, which was made for pedestrians, you'll find what I call 3-miles-an-hour architectural. Everything is detailed and scaled in such a way that you have a glorious time moving at 3 miles per hour. All the old cities would have the 3 miles per hour scale.

*(Source: Sierra Club interview, January 29, 2010 http://sierraclub.typepad.com/greenlife/2010/01/ architect-jan-gehls-bicycle-revolution-.html)*

a previous century are all legible. I can actually stop, read and learn something about the history of my city. This makes me feel more connected to the place and the people who came before me.

In particular, I find that walking allows for chance conversations with people who know a place's story — talking with them is better than learning from a history book or a description of a monument. Walking around Savannah, I've met and talked with people who have lived here for decades and told me wonderful anecdotes about the city. They know what was in a particular building, who did something important in a certain square, and generally what life was like in previous eras. On one fall day last year, I noticed an older man walking slowly around a square as he was leaving church. We said "hello," and then began to chat in a friendly way. He described for me in great detail some of his experiences as a child growing up in the neighborhood many decades ago and changes in the area, such as the bank that used be on the corner and the drugstore opposite. He described how different life was then, in both good ways and bad.

Such encounters help me understand the city, and they enrich my life. This type of interaction is something I wouldn't get locked up in my car, rushing to the next strip mall or drive-through.

## I learn more about people.

I'm an architect, so at times I tend to focus first on how walking helps me interact with buildings and places before I discuss interaction with people. We all end up fitting some stereotypes!

By far, the most important connections that walking facilitates are those with other humans, as I began discussing above. The vast majority of the time, such interactions are silent. We walk by each other, perhaps smile, and continue on our ways. But, because I walk most everywhere, on a regular basis something else happens. I actually speak with people!

I may learn about the city, as mentioned, or I may learn about the person. What I learn could be something seemingly minor, such as something that is readily apparent about the person. Perhaps it's that he or she obviously likes bright clothes, or obviously is a people person, or obviously had a bad day. The list is endless, since the behavior of human beings is so endlessly unpredictable.

Or what I learn might not be something obvious. I might interact with someone who is different from me in some significant way. That person might be poorer, wealthier, louder, quieter or just plain out of their head. The reality is, when we walk around in public, we get the chance to see, hear and smell all of humanity. And by that I mean *all* of humanity: the good, the bad and the bizarre.

I understand that this type of interaction is not for everyone. Many people prefer to surround themselves with others who either look like them, are of the same income group, or the same age. We find no shortage of ways to self-segregate in a free society.

When I drove all the time, I never had these kinds of interactions with people. My chance interactions were through the

## Your Dog Can Introduce You

It's no secret that dog walking is a surprisingly effective method for meeting people. The presence of a dog tends to soften up complete strangers, including ones who may at first seem unapproachable. If you're looking to meet people, get a dog. You can maximize the dog's effectiveness when you stroll in an already walkable environment, as opposed to driving to a dog park next to the highway.

There's a fascinating recent BBC documentary, *Walking with Dogs: a Wonderland Special,* about people walking their dogs in London and the intimate conversations among strangers that the presence of dogs seems to facilitate (Find it at http://www.telegraph.co.uk/culture/tvandradio/9605610/Vanessa-Engle-Im-amazed-how-honest-people-are-about-their-lives.html or https://www.youtube.com/watch?v+8-EOrOpus for full length documentary.)

closed windows of my car or maybe with the windows down, if I got lucky. I'm talking about interactions such as the occasional smile or wave, but frequently it was an angry look or upraised middle finger.

Today, not all of my interactions while walking are shiny and happy ones by any means. But more often than not, something happens that makes me smile or think, instead of making me hit the gas pedal harder.

### Make Walking & Biking Easy Tip 7:
*Have Comfortable Shoes — Seriously*

This isn't just a tip for the ladies out there. If you walk a lot, shoes matter. If you can find style and comfort, go for it. If not, go for comfort. Your feet and back will thank you, and it's perhaps the most important step you can take to encourage regular walking.

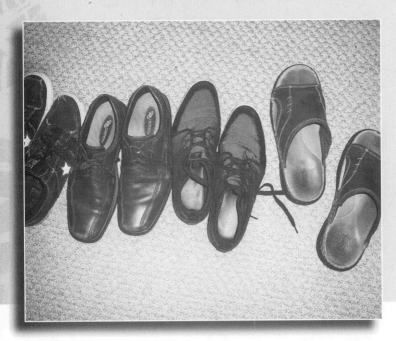

> I don't have to move out of my neighborhood as my wants, needs and circumstances change.

It's inevitable that as we move through life, what we want out of a home or a neighborhood changes. As a young adult, I want-ed to rent somewhere cool and cheap and didn't care about much else. Later, I wanted a little more room to call my own. When I added dogs to my life, I really wanted a small yard for them, and for me, frankly. People have kids, get married, get divorced, get older, etc. The point is, we rarely stay in the same house or apartment for more than five or ten years.

The downside to moving so much is that we often feel we have to move to an entirely new neighborhood if we're staying in the same city in order to accommodate our evolving require-ments. So many subdivisions and communities are filled with the identical house or apartment for block after block that when what we want in our living space changes, we have to look far-ther afield for something different. If we've made good friends where we are, moving means leaving them behind to some de-gree and putting a strain on social bonds that we may enjoy.

In a walkable neighborhood, a change in housing require-ments (or desires) manifests itself differently. A well-planned

## Americans on the Move

It's an article of faith that Americans move more often than just about anyone else in the world. Data from the Census Bureau backs this up. Americans move on average fourteen times in their lifetimes, compared to five times in Great Britain and four times in Japan. Approximately forty million Americans move every year.

(*Source: http://voices.yahoo.com/census-bureau-report-americans-move-too-much-2983301. html?cat=7//*)

and well-built walkable place has a wide mixture of kinds of houses, condos and apartments. This is part of the nature of more compact neighborhoods. If I like a particular pedestrian-friendly neighborhood, I can probably find something that suits whatever phase of life I'm in.

In my two and a half years in Savannah, I've lived in three rented apartments of various sizes and designs within just a few blocks of each other. Should I choose to purchase a home, the same area has townhouses and condos for sale, as well as a wide range of single-family houses. Should I reach my golden years here, there's even some senior housing in the neighborhood.

Why do I care about staying in a neighborhood? I care because those social bonds that I forge in one place can continue to build over time. I won't lose friends simply because I get older or married or divorced or have children — because I won't need to relocate to accommodate different housing requirements. Of course, you can always keep friends no matter where you and

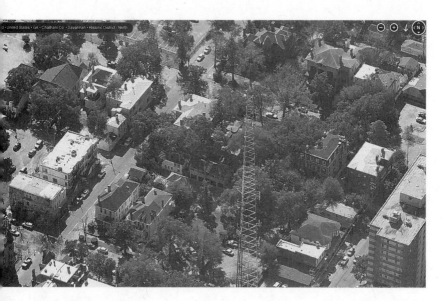

*Something for everyone.*

they are, and today's technology makes it easier. But it's also true that we tend to have the strongest social bonds with the people we see and interact with the most often. Proximity still matters for most relationships.

The bottom line is that I have more options in a walkable place. I may *want* to move away from long-time social contacts, but I don't *have* to. I may *want* to move into a different neighborhood or part of town, but I don't *have* to. The choices are mine, not forced upon me.

## I won't be confined to being around only old people as I age.

There's a strain of housing development unique to the United States called *age-restricted*. You know these places — Sun City, del Boca Vista Phase 3, the Villages, and so on. These are places for *Active Adults,* or *fifty-five-plus,* or *able-bodied retirees enjoying their golden years* — in other words, retirement communities.

These are developments that have filled a niche. As we've become more and more mobile as a society (thanks to our cars), we've increasingly formed communities based on the phase of life we're in. We have an apartment or rental community when we're young, a starter home community for that first house, and a move-up community for when we need more house and yard. Then, when the kids are gone, we head towards the fifty-five-plus, or age-restricted, places. The market has nimbly responded to how we've separated our communities out into so many different pods.

But our communities don't have to be segregated in this way. We lose something very important socially when people hit a certain age and are practically expected to move to a different part of town or even a different state. In the previous section, I noted how in my neighborhood I have a variety of housing options available, so I don't have to leave as my needs change. For

## JARGON ALERT: *Active Adult*

You have to love the terms the housing industry comes up with. Did you know houses are referred to as *product*? In the never-ending process to come up with new terms for "senior housing" or "retirement communities," the housing industry came up with *Active Adult*. I suppose that is something different from Inactive Adults. At any rate, *Active Adult Communities* are specifically designed for people age fifty-five and up.

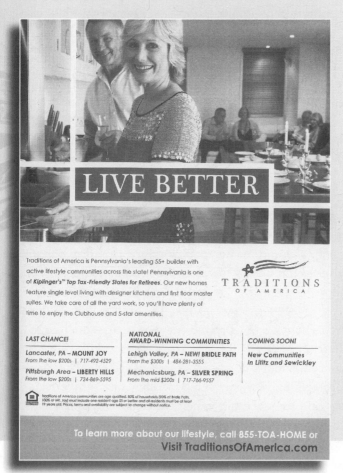

*What is a Mature Adult anyway?*

# 8 / DYNAMIC LOCALES TO FIND WALKABLE LIVING

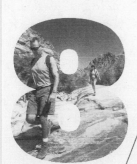

More people than ever are making retirement relocation decisions based in part on how often they can ditch the car and go places by foot.

> By Julie Fanselow

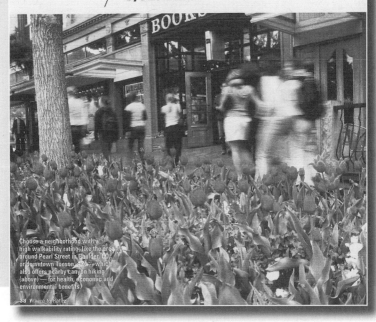

Choose a neighborhood with a high walkability rating, like the area around Pearl Street in Boulder, CO, or downtown Tucson, AZ — which also offers nearby canyon hiking (above) — for health, economic and environmental benefits.

38 Where to Retire

122 Why I Walk

me, that's a big deal, because I, for one, don't like living where I'm surrounded by people who are all just like me, or all the same age as me.

Hopefully, all of us will get to experience old age. I know that if I reach my senior years, the last thing I will want is to be surrounded by only other old people. I can't imagine anything more depressing and confining. Golf course communities and early-bird specials? No thanks.

This age diversity isn't just something that will be important to me later on — it matters to me now, in my forties. The daily sights and sounds of people younger than me enhance my life immeasurably. Seeing young kids, college students and young professionals keeps my mind more engaged and active. How boring would it be if I only got to see and hang out with people my own age all the time?

## I never have to worry about drinking and driving.

Let's face it — we humans like to imbibe. Wine, beer, whiskey and other liquors fill our homes, our restaurants, our bars, our

### Make Walking & Biking Easy Tip 8:
### *Text Your Cab Company or Use an App*
I'm fully expecting and looking forward to the day that taxis will be much more automated and even driverless. In the meantime, some cab companies are finally adopting better methods for working with customers. In many places, you can now text a cab company for a pick-up. Some progressive companies have their own apps that make the process easier. In any case, if you think you'll need a cab frequently, it's a good idea to build a relationship with a reliable cabby or cab company. Trust me, it will come in handy.

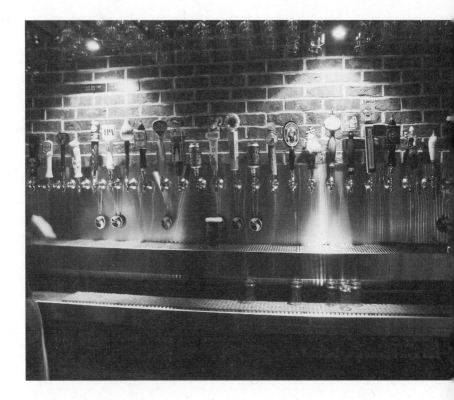

*Life is too short to drink cheap beer.*

festivals, our holidays, etc. There's nothing wrong with that —
it's part of our lives, and I'm not alone in enjoying a few drinks.
I'm a big fan of craft beers, good wine and classic cocktails, either
with a meal or without.

But there is a problem unique to American cities and towns
related to alcohol, and it's directly connected to our acceptance
of driving to almost all of our destinations. That problem is our
proclivity to get behind the wheel of a car and drive after drinking. It's a dangerous and foolish thing to do, and I'm not too
proud to admit I've done it myself. For most of my life, I've lived
in cities where driving was the only realistic way to get around,
and I've succumbed to the stupid impulse to drive myself home

## Are You Impaired?

No chart can perfectly define drunkenness or ascertain ability to drive. The many factors include sex, weight, genetics, type of drink, length of time drinking, etc. A good rule of thumb is that two standard drinks in the first hour will have you approaching the legal limit for blood alcohol content. You can find many more comprehensive charts by searching the Internet. One in particular that I think is very good is this link: http://www.brad21.org/bac_charts.html

when I shouldn't have. Luckily for me and everyone else, none of the worst-case scenarios have happened. But I repeat: I've been lucky.

Alcohol and drug abuse are complex, touchy subjects, as is drinking and driving. People are seriously injured or killed by drunk drivers all too often. It's such a pervasive problem in American society that we are barraged with advertising messages warning us against it. And there are constantly evolving strategies and tactics designed to reduce the incidence of drunk driving, including tougher and tougher DUI laws, frequent sobriety checkpoints and more readily available "Tipsy Taxis" at special events.

The problem is that no amount of MADD commercials or creative strategies will eradicate people's desire to drink — and they certainly won't overcome our spread-out cities. In my experience, only one approach can solve the problem, and that's living in a place where you don't have to drive.

In my living situation, I can drink as much as I like and not have to worry about consequences — except to my own liver and the potential for embarrassment. Living in a pedestrian-friendly place means I can walk home after having some drinks or take a cheap taxi, as I'm close enough to make the fare home inexpensive. I'm never a threat to anyone else or to myself.

I find this aspect of living in a walkable place to be a great emotional relief. "Who will be the designated driver?" is a question that never has to come up, nor does the accompanying awkwardness and lack of fun. I get to relax and enjoy myself instead of running a blood-alcohol-content (BAC) calculation in my head while I'm out. Even better, I don't have to play nanny to anyone else I'm with to monitor his or her BAC. I also don't have to crash uncomfortably on a friend's couch because I've had too much to drink.

Think about that feeling you have when you're on vacation somewhere very relaxing and walkable. You find yourself often strolling over to a bar or restaurant to have a few drinks. Afterwards, you likely stumble back to your room and sleep the night away. We all do this time and again, then get home and marvel at how relaxing the vacation was. All the while, it never crosses our mind that one major reason it was so relaxing was because driving was not an issue. At home, we meet friends for a happy hour but cut the fun short because we have to drive. How much more relaxing is that glass of wine, knowing we don't have to get in a car and drive home? And how much safer is it for everyone? Why do we settle for that carefree attitude only on vacation?

## Drinking and Driving: The Numbers

Alcohol-related fatalities are about half of what they were in the early 1980s, which indicates that the increased awareness is having an impact. Still, over ten thousand people per year are killed in drunk driving accidents in the US, which is far too many. In 2010, over 1.4 million people were arrested for driving under the influence of alcohol or narcotics.

*(Source: Centers for Disease Control and Prevention http://www.cdc.gov/motorvehiclesafety/ impaired_driving/impaired-drv_factsheet.html///).*

## I don't need a lawn mower or a big yard.

Lawn care is not my thing. I know: it's heresy for an American man to admit this. But it's true. The last thing I want to spend my time doing is endless hours of yard work. It's pure drudgery for me, and when I do it, all I can think about is what else I'd rather be doing.

There are too many people like me who don't like lawn care but have chosen to live in a way that makes it a required chore. We tend to have big yards that need care because we think we have to have them. We dedicate weekend and leisure time to something we, at best, tolerate. At every opportunity, we look for someone else to pick up the slack. Can the kids mow the lawn? The neighbor kid? Parents? A landscape company?

I know there are a sick and twisted few who love lawn care. They live for the riding lawn mower, the edger, the seeding and weeding, and the hours of worry about whether the grass is getting enough water. Count me out.

My lack of desire to have or maintain a yard doesn't mean I don't want and need beautiful and usable landscapes in my life. To the contrary, I think as humans we all crave some form of regular time in nature, and we love getting our hands dirty every once in a while.

So how do I reconcile these competing urges with my lifestyle choice?

First, even though I don't like lawns, I do like gardens. Whether it's growing some simple flowering bushes, or having my own vegetables, I do find it rewarding to put whatever small slice of land I have to productive use. It not only can add beauty, but also can provide me with something useful: fresh food. This year, in a very small piece of sandy earth, I'll be growing some tomatoes, onions, cilantro and jalapeno peppers. I won't win any farm-to-table awards, but I will have some cheap, tasty food to eat this summer.

Second, when I need a bigger hit of "green," I have parks nearby. Whether they are small squares or large city parks, I have access to expanses of trees, flowers and lawns within an

## Would You Rather Care for a Lawn or Enjoy Your life?

An article from *USA Today* about the new renting economy highlighted how people's attitudes are changing about yard work and even home-ownership. Here's an excerpt:

> The Jacobsons aren't so wistful about home ownership.
>
> For the past 19 months, they've rented in The Arbors. Their home is neat and clean, their furnishings are fashionable. Yet, their backyard is 200 square feet of dirt and weeds, just as it was when they moved in. They keep the shades drawn.
>
> Instead of paying $2,100 on a monthly mortgage payment, they pay $1,243.38 to rent. Instead of spending weekends fixing up their home, they go to an occasional jazz club.
>
> "I guess that was fun," says Jodi Jacobson, 38, when recalling the weekends spent at their former home. "But do we have any vacation memories from that time? No." Since their foreclosure, they've taken one vacation. They expect to take more.
>
> If they ever buy a home again, they say they'll buy something smaller. "I would never put so much of my income again into a house," Steve Jacobson says.

*(Source: "Home rentals — the new American dream?" USA Today, June 5, 2012 http://usatoday30. usatoday.com/money/economy/housing/story/2012-06-05/are-home-rentals-the-new- american-dream/55402648/1.)*

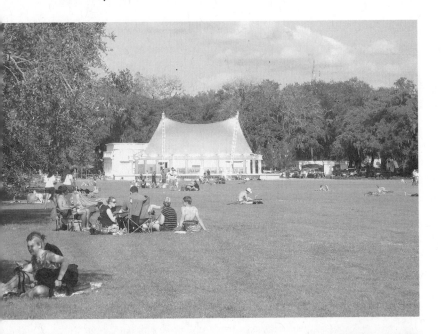

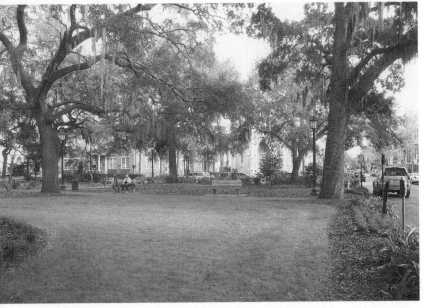

*My backyard.*

easy walk. These places do so much more for me than any toil in the backyard ever could. Not only are they big enough to spread out in and enjoy in a wide variety of ways, but I don't have to take care of them myself.

Not all neighborhoods have as much quality public space as what I have available to me in Savannah. I'm lucky in that sense. But it's not an accident that I live here — the public spaces were one important reason why I chose to live in this particular city. Unfortunately, many of our cities (of all sizes) are in desperate need of better located and better designed parks and squares. Having this green space nearby and easily accessible makes the big backyard something I never miss.

## My trash is better looking than your trash.

I'm a guy. So, apparently trash is my lifelong responsibility.

I can't stand the weekly mess that appears in the streets of so many places. It's a bit of my own personal OCD. We put the trash out in front of the house for everyone to see. If we're lucky, the trash haulers actually get all of it into the truck, rather than leaving portions of it scattered on the ground. In my experience, getting that lucky is a rarity. Instead, in most of the places I've lived, my neighbors and I frequently battled trash of all kinds strewn around the fronts of our homes. Having debris littering the ground is not just a pain, it's also a blight.

In the best walkable places, the residences have alleys in back where the trash receptacles are kept. Alleys (or "lanes," as they are called here, and elsewhere in the South) are a much better and more attractive way to deal with trash and recycling; the bins and containers are out of sight and don't clutter up the street. I'm far less likely to be concerned about the appearance of the back of my property than the front, since very few people actually see the back. And likewise, I'm not as concerned with

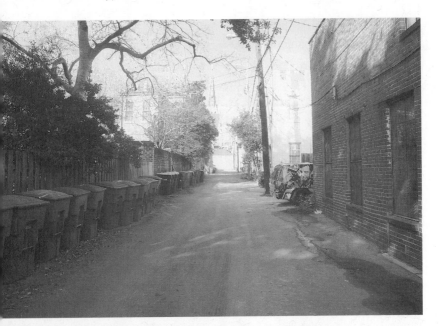

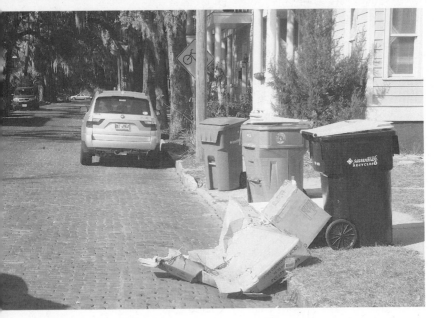

*Where should the trash go?*

what I see of my neighbors out the back, as opposed to what can be seen out the front door.

This distinction between front and back, or public and private, is part of what has changed over the years in terms of how we build our cities. We used to have buildings with a clear front that was public and a clear back that was private and quiet. People mostly walked to get where they were going, so the relationship between the front door (and front porch, if there was one) and the street was very important. Think for a moment of the scene from *It's a Wonderful Life* when George Bailey walks by Mary's house, and she has a conversation with him from her window. It's a small but fantastic illustration of how much more public our lives were when we used to walk routinely. And since our lives were much more on display, that distinction between public and private was extremely significant. Everything from the front door of the house through the back was designed with public versus private in mind. The more public the front became, the more private the back needed to be, to give us a way to balance our human needs for both private time and sociability.

As we adopted the car culture, we shifted this arrangement of front and back, public and private. The front of our homes became like the alleys of old — the front is something we essentially *drive* into, entering our garages with our cars. The back has become our semi-private space, with big lawns and usually fences between yards. Instead of socializing in the front and having private gatherings in the back, we shifted to socializing on the back patio, deck or yard and having private gatherings inside the house.

This front-back relationship has impacted every aspect of our lives, including the topic of this section: trash. In previous eras, the notion that people would display all of their garbage in front of their houses would have been inconceivable — it would have been considered unseemly. Trash obviously belonged in the back, in a more private, hidden spot. As with trash, the trucks themselves were largely unseen, being relegated to the alleys rather than cluttering up our streets.

In most places, that's all changed. We now put our colored bins, our recycling, our bags of leaves, our old furniture and so much more out front for the world to see. It's an element of ugliness that we've come to accept as normal. But in some walkable places, we still have alleys that can handle garbage and recycling trucks, which leaves our fronts a little more well-kept. For me, getting the trash out of sight has a positive impact on my quality of life. For society at large, the changing nature of where we put our trash is a classic example of how changing to accommodate cars has affected so many details of our daily lives.

## JARGON ALERT: *Front-Back Relationship*

Architects love to talk about how buildings have a relationship with the street. What's the nature of this relationship? Is it monogamous? Open? No, it's actually the much more boring notion that a building should have its entry in an obvious location vis-à-vis the street (or sidewalk), and it should appear to have "open arms" toward the public. A good reason for this configuration is that traditionally the front contains the more "public" rooms of a house, such as the foyer, living room, etc. The back of a house is better suited for more private spaces. Such was the way we designed and built for centuries, until we started designing our streets primarily for cars. Since then, our houses have taken on a huge variety of configurations. We have master bedrooms at the front of the house, and living rooms in back. We have great rooms that open to all directions, and public spaces in basements. The front-back relationship from an earlier time is no longer.

## Walking on vacation.

My parents infected me with the travel bug at a young age. There's nothing I enjoy more than getting to a place I have never visited and going out to explore. On foot, of course.

The funny thing about vacationing is that we typically spend our hard-earned dollars going to places where we get around primarily on foot. Fifty weeks out of the year we work hard, scrimp and save, and spend hours sitting in traffic so we can spend two weeks somewhere in Europe or Mexico or New York or Disneyworld where we can . . . walk.

When on vacation we walk, we live a bit slower, and we find ourselves enjoying the day just a little more. Sure, some of that is because we don't have the pressures of the daily grind. But how much of our enjoyment is because we have a completely different kind of experience getting around? Instead of sitting in a car and traffic, we use our own bodies to explore the world around us. My sense is that quite a bit of our happiness on vacation stems from being on foot.

So why don't we just choose to live in places where we can do this all the time?

But I digress.

I'm famous in my family for taking everyone on extended walks when we're together on vacation. "It's just up around the corner" in my language means it's several more blocks. "We're

### Great Walks in Europe

The *New York Times* ran this beautiful piece in 2013 about nine great walks in Europe. Check out "Europe in Nine Walks" at nytimes.com http://travel.nytimes.com/2013/04/21/travel/europe-in-9-walks.html.

almost there" means we've got about another ten minutes to go. My family thinks I have a different meter for distance and walking than what normal people do.

When on vacation, I can jump right into walking and spending the days out and about because of how I live my life when I'm home. Because I'm used to walking on a daily basis, it's no big deal for me to walk long distances when I'm on vacation. And, as with being at home, walking while on vacation means I get to see so much of a place up close and personally.

Walking adds to my pleasure on vacations and allows me to get to know an unfamiliar place much more quickly. If you're not used to walking and have to limit yourself while on vacation, your experience and interaction with that place and its people becomes far different and, in my opinion, less rich.

## Walking in America's Tourist Hotspots

Here's a list of the most-visited tourist destinations in the United States. Note that nearly all of these are places where people get around primarily by walking.

- New York City
- Las Vegas
- Washington, DC
- Boston
- Disneyworld
- Disneyland
- San Francisco
- Niagara Falls
- Smoky Mountains
- Chicago

(Source: Forbes Traveler Magazine *http://www.thetravelerszone.com/travel-destinations/top-25-most-visited-tourist-destinations-in-america/*)

## Vacation Stroll

*Walk, Forrest, Walk!*

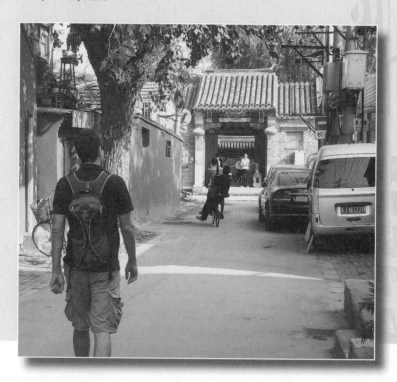

Walking regularly is one of those activities that is truly self-reinforcing. The more of it I do, the more I like to do. The less I do — which may happen if I'm on a work trip and in a location that isn't conducive to walking — the harder it becomes to motivate myself to walk at all.

So take that long walk on vacation. Enjoy the sights and sounds at a slow pace. Imagine doing the same in your own town. Then do it, and you'll no doubt find yourself walking longer distances in no time. Better yet, you'll develop a greater appreciation for your own surroundings.

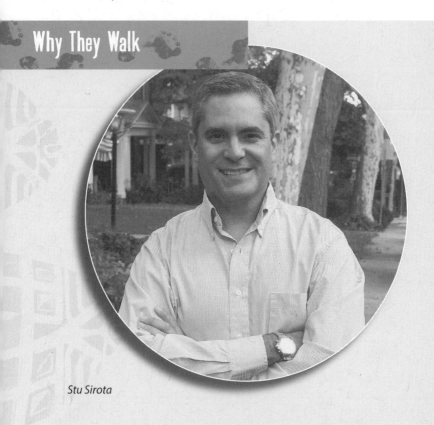

*Stu Sirota*

I left my former auto-dependent life behind for good in January, 2002 and have never looked back. It began when I sold my 1963 ranch house located in the Levitt-built suburb of Bowie, Maryland (Walk Score: 13). Walk Score is a website that ranks a place's walk-ability. It was the first home I ever owned, and I lived in it for nearly twelve years. In its place, I bought a classic Baltimore rowhouse with white marble steps, built in 1898, in the heart of the historic Riverside Park neighborhood (Walk Score: 87).

I made the move to this gentrifying, up-and-coming neighborhood when my wife was expecting our first child. The move from suburb to city allowed me to trade in my fifty-minute (each way) daily driving commute for a twenty-minute walking commute. Doing so not only dramatically reduced my overall commute time but also provided me new choices for how to get to work, including taking the bus (a door-to-door ten-minute ride) or a five-minute taxicab ride. It also made me feel good to know that I was no longer polluting the environment and was becoming healthier in the process.

The daily walk to work into the heart of downtown Baltimore was truly a transformative experience that provided a new and radically different way of interacting with my world. The walk took me down lovely, charming streets of Federal Hill, past the historic Cross Street Market, through the famous Inner Harbor waterfront, and into Baltimore's central business district where I worked in a high-rise office tower. When arriving at work, I no longer found myself feeling stressed out and irritable, as I often did when I commuted by car. Rather, I felt energized and relaxed. On the trip home, I often found myself spontaneously walking through the block-long Cross Street Market building and picking up fresh meat, produce, desserts and flowers. No parking required. This new lifestyle also made owning two cars completely unnecessary, so we downsized to just one vehicle without any sacrifice in convenience. In the process, we also quickly realized that this change was saving us over $8,000 annually.

Several years and two kids later, we decided to sell the small city home we had outgrown and move to a bigger house in a more family-friendly neighborhood with better public schools. Not wanting to give up our car-independence, we decided on a walkable neighborhood just outside of Baltimore City in the prewar "streetcar suburb" of Rodgers Forge, consisting of much larger stately rowhouses (Walk Score: 67). What drew us to this location was its walkability, combined with beautiful, tree-lined streets and the presence of a highly acclaimed public elementary school located in the heart of the neighborhood and less than a ten-minute walk away.

During this period, I decided to quit my job and start my own consulting firm, which eliminated the need for me to commute downtown. For the last three years I have leased a suite in a small office building at the end of my street, a mere five-minute walk from home.

My wife has been a stay-at-home mom for the last ten years, and between the two of us, now with three kids, we still have just one vehicle that gets driven lightly each year. On the rare occasion that we both need a car at the same time, I rent a car for the day from nearby Enterprise or opt for a Zipcar for a few hours via a five-minute bike ride to the local college campus. We walk our three kids to school most of the time, and many of our errands are within walking distance.

We've found that the walkable living arrangement we have created for ourselves is deeply satisfying. It affords us a great deal of convenience and choice while allowing us to live in a close-knit neighborhood where we know our neighbors and look out for each other. Walkability provides us a feeling of resilience and less vulnerability to potential energy disruptions or even natural disasters than those living in car-dependent areas. We also feel like we are "part of the solution" from an environmental standpoint, in that our carbon footprint is probably less than one-fifth that of the average American household of five.

I can't imagine ever living anywhere again that would take us back to a car-dependent living arrangement. Doing so would greatly reduce our quality of life as well as our sense of security and well-being.

— Stuart Sirota
Baltimore, MD

# 4<sup>th</sup> Interlude — *Far beyond a simple stroll*

Some places are either too far to walk, or too unpleasant of a walk to draw me there on foot. But, they still require a trip occasionally. Here's a few.

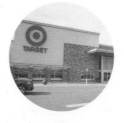

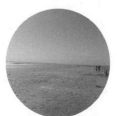

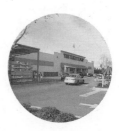

Yep, we all go to
these stores

Home improvement,
hardware, you name it

The Mall

What's remaining of
electronics stores

The multiplex

Ah, the beach

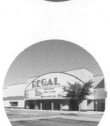

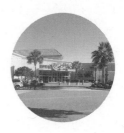

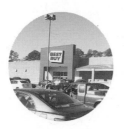

There's a long line of cars
And they're trying to get through
There's no single explanation
There's no central destination
But this long line of cars
Is trying to get through
And this long line of cars
Is all because of you
You don't wonder where we're going
Or remember where we've been
We've got to keep this traffic
Flowing and accept a little spin
So this long line of cars
will never have an end
And this long line of cars
Keeps coming around the bend
From the streets of Sacramento
To the freeways of L.A.
We've got to keep this fire burning
and accept a little gray
So this long line of cars
Is trying to break free
And this long line of cars
Is all because of me

— Cake lyrics, "Long Line of Cars"

# 6

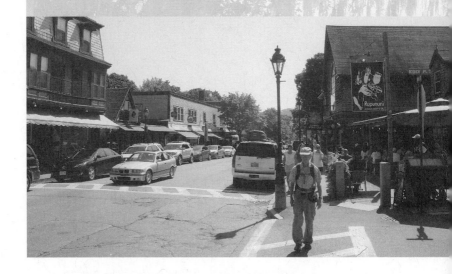

## *Caveat Emptor*: There Are Some Downsides

'Cause on the surface the city lights shine
They're calling at me, come and find your kind
Sometimes I wonder if the World's so small
That we can never get away from the sprawl
Living in the sprawl
Dead shopping malls rise like mountains beyond
mountains
And there's no end in sight
I need the darkness, someone please cut the lights

— Arcade Fire lyrics
"Sprawl II: Mountains Beyond Mountains"

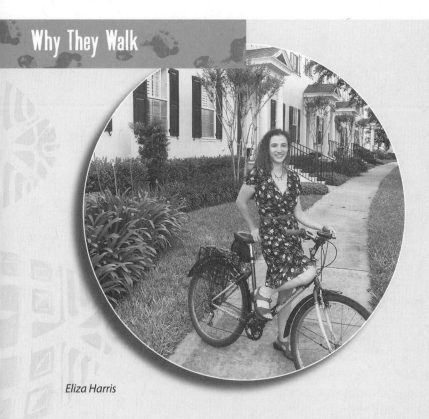

*Eliza Harris*

I bike to work nearly every day. I also bike nearly everywhere else. I always get the best parking spot, and it's always free. Sometimes a few of us just ride around the grid all evening from a restaurant to a bar to a park and then maybe to a friend's house to sit around the fire pit or watch a movie.

It's even a lovely walk to work. It takes about forty minutes. I've done this a few times when my bike was in the shop or I was carpooling somewhere after work. I can also walk to my bike shop and my auto mechanic, so I don't have to contend with rides, taxis or shuttles when it's time for an oil change or an overhaul. When my car is in the shop, I usually tell them to take their time; I don't have to drive anywhere until next week anyway. Whether I walk, bike or drive, I can take quiet, tree-lined streets. The interstate seems rather harrowing by comparison; I swear I can feel my blood pressure go up with the stop-go, stop-go.

People often ask me if I own a car because they don't know what it looks like. Sometimes I have to drive it just to make sure it still works. I'm constantly surprised by gas prices. I only fill up every month or two, and that's usually because I'm making the six-hour drive to my hometown or heading out to a state park to go hiking or biking. So every time I do show up at the pump, the change seems rather dramatic. I'm not the proverbial frog in boiling water anymore. I finally lost that freshman fifteen, too (better late than never!). In fact, I think I might fit into my prom dress if I bothered to get it out of the plastic.

Last Thursday, my book club showed up for our weekly meeting at a member's house with no chapter assigned. So we decided to find a place for dinner. Most of us decided to walk. Along the way, we talked and laughed and shuffled partners and conversations. One person had to drive because he was meeting a friend afterwards, so a few of the guys piled into his car. We saw them walk in about a minute before us. We poked fun because the guys were the ones complaining about the "cold" Florida weather. After dinner, the driver went to meet his friend, and the rest of us (including the carpoolers) all walked back together. One of the women said, "This is so different. I never really walk to places. This was actually kind of nice."

— Eliza Harris
Orlando, FL

I'm not saying that once you lace up your walking shoes and head out the door, it's all roses and puppies. Choosing to live in a walkable place does present some difficulties and obstacles, as do all choices. I've outlined the benefits as I see them. But to be fair, here are a few of the problematic issues that you may encounter if you to choose to live a walking lifestyle.

### There aren't enough walkable places.

This is unfortunate, but true. We have far too few places where someone can get around primarily by walking and biking and live a full and complete life. This limited supply problem not only makes choosing a walkable place more difficult, it also creates a supply/demand imbalance that makes housing more expensive than it should be. In today's market, housing is generally more expensive in the quality walkable places than it is elsewhere. Only time and a whole lot more supply will ultimately tip this imbalance to the consumer's favor.

### Our workplaces are scattered far and wide.

As a consequence, many people have to drive long distances to get to their jobs. As long as our cities and suburbs are so spread out, we will continue to have this problem. While more of us are working from home or have a flexible work arrangement that allows us to work from home at least part of the time, most people still have to commute to work. We need better planning in our cities so that workplaces aren't as spread out and so people have options when it comes to transportation, such as taking an efficient train or bus.

### Too many of the best shopping options are located in far-away areas that require a car to get there.

Shopping malls, while not as ubiquitous as they used to be, still contain a lot of our stores and often are nowhere near an easy walking or transit trip. The same is true for the popular, inexpensive big-box stores. Target, Walmart, Best Buy, Kohl's, you name it — they are not easy to get to without a car, and it's certainly not easy to take home all that cheap stuff if you don't have a car to put it in. Online shopping and services like car sharing can be useful work-arounds for this situation, but the far-flung locations of our stores is still an inconvenience of daily life.

### Schools in many walkable places aren't good.

The problem of school quality isn't due to neighborhood design, but stems from our legacy of racial and social issues. Even worse, schools are sometimes nonexistent in walkable places because they've either been closed or consolidated. This needs to change. The lack of good schools keeps many families with young kids from living in walkable places. In addition, the ability to walk to school should be a given for any kid.

### Crime and safety are real issues.

Regardless of statistics, the cocoon of a car provides a tremendous psychological sense of protection for people concerned about their safety. We sometimes feel safer just knowing that our car is parked out there somewhere. When we're walking, especially late at night when it's dark, our vulnerability meter goes way up. For women especially, this is a real concern. As a man, I rarely feel worried about my safety when walking. But there are times that it can feel creepy, for lack of a better word, even to me. There's no question our cities need better and more effective policing. We need to get our policemen and -women who work in walkable places to step out of their cars and patrol on foot, bike, horse or whatever. We know this kind of patrolling is more effective, and it can become the important security blanket to help get people out and about more often. In the case of walkable areas and safety, more people are definitely better.

# Getting Cops Out of Their Cars

Peter Moskos wrote about his year as a police officer in Baltimore in the book *Cop in the Hood: My Year Policing Baltimore's Eastern District*. Here's what he wrote in the Afterword about the virtues of patrolling on foot instead of in cars:

> Foot patrol used to define policing, and even today a certain romantic stereotype of the espantoon-twirling beat cop persists. But by and large when police start driving, they never walk on foot again. That's a shame. Foot patrol officers know the neighborhood and see more than officers in cars do. The key to foot patrol's success, especially in maintaining order and seeing and stopping potential crimes before they start, is long-term presence and building knowledge of the community. The beat cop watched people grow up, get jobs, or get in trouble. It's much better to see and understand a small area well than a large area not at all. Think of the difference between a group of residents enjoying themselves on a stoop and the same group of people causing trouble; it's subtle but immediately apparent to anybody walking by. In a car, you simply can't see.

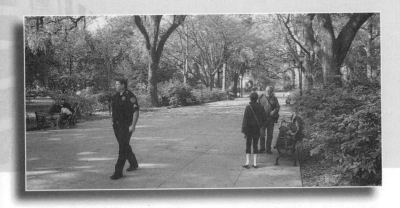

### *Our walking and biking infrastructure needs a lot of improvement.*

Obviously, I love walking and biking to get around. But I also put up with a lot of obstacles that I shouldn't have to put up with. Our neighborhoods have far too many incomplete sidewalks, streets without shade and little or no thought given to pedestrians. Our planning for bikes is even worse. We need much better bike lanes that truly protect riders from moving cars and more bike parking and bike sharing programs. As we fell in love with the car culture, we retrofitted our cities far too much for cars, in the form of wide roads, one-way streets, freeways barreling through neighborhoods and buildings torn down for parking. It's time to correct those mistakes and stitch our places back together.

### *Noise can be an issue.*

People generally worry too much about how noisy life can be in a compact place. In fact, the streets are often far quieter, especially at night, than most people assume. Even living in close proximity to others, noise is not an issue the majority of the time. I have found that I even have become immune to a certain amount of background noise. But there are times when it *does* get noisy. Housing in a compact place often means living in apartments or attached buildings. Sharing walls and/or floors puts you into close contact with people — and their noise. Additionally, the narrow streets found in walkable places causes sound to reverberate more. This isn't always a bad thing, but if you're sensitive to noise, it may be a problem for you.

### *Some people can be really obnoxious.*

Whether it's bad manners, drunken parties, or aggressive behavior, you get to deal with all kinds of people when you live in a walkable, compact place. Of course this isn't all bad. Most people are generally good people, and you get to form relationships

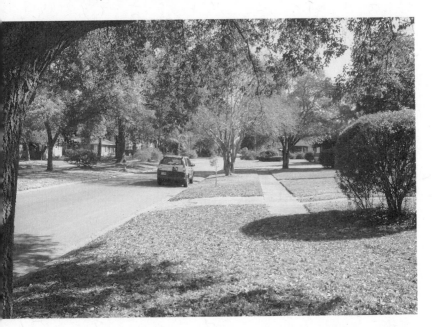

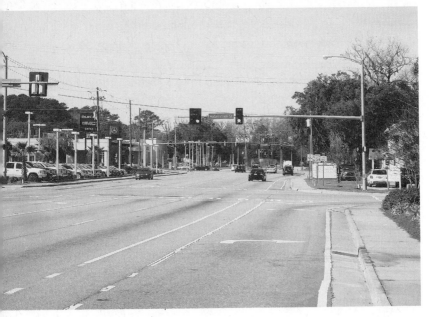

*Sidewalks and bike lanes that aren't useful.*

with them. And, you also learn street smarts pretty quickly. But some people can be real assholes, and it's harder to escape them when you live in close proximity to lots of people. It's a potential downside to this way of life, and one you have to learn how to deal with.

### I have to relearn how to dress for the weather.

Now admittedly, this is not too big of a deal for me. Being out and about means I have to remember to bundle up when it's cold and wear the right clothing when it's hot and humid. But for women, dressing for the weather is more of an issue. Anyone who is concerned about how they look when they leave their home as well as how they *might* look after walking for fifteen minutes in rainy/cold/humid weather has to put more thought and effort into choosing the right clothes. While our predecessors used to dress for the weather as a matter of course, we have gotten out of the habit, growing up in a time when cars have made it easy for us to ignore the weather. You can't ignore the weather if you walk and bike a lot.

### Our city zoning rules are too restrictive.

I know more about zoning issues than most people, since I work with cities on zoning codes. But you don't have to be an expert in zoning codes to understand what I mean. All you need is to spend some time living in one of these places. Almost every good walkable place was built before we had much in the way of rules for building and zoning. As a result, walkable places have a much wider mixture of types of buildings and uses of buildings than what we typically allow today. As cities have updated their rules, they've done so in ways that are now too tough on the good things that make places work well. Too many codes don't allow for carriage houses, corner stores, home occupations, or apartments or residences over shops. In a walkable place, it's all about the mix. And more of the mix is generally good.

***Even in good places, we have too many bad buildings.***
As an architect, I can't resist including this pet peeve. The buildings I refer to are "bad" for varied reasons: they may have been built poorly, with little design thought, or set back behind a parking lot, or be out of character with the neighborhood, or just generally not feel "local." The noted twentieth-century architect and town planner Trystan Edwards would call this "bad manners in architecture." Our cities have endured a lot of wrong-headed "improvements" and "renewals" over the last few decades. I'm a big fan of removing the eyesores that hurt our places and healing them with good buildings. After all, good buildings make for good walks.

# Epilogue: What You Can Do

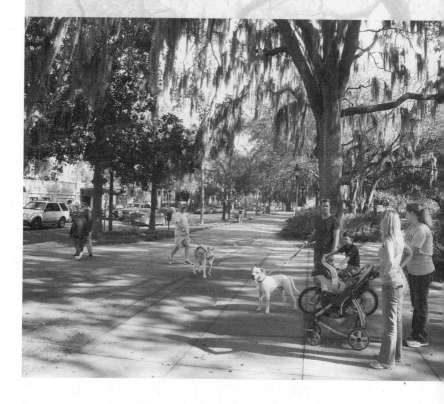

*I would walk along the quais when I had finished work or when I was trying to think something out. It was easier to think if I was walking and doing something or seeing people doing something that they understood.*

— Ernest Hemingway, *A Moveable Feast*

# Why They Walk

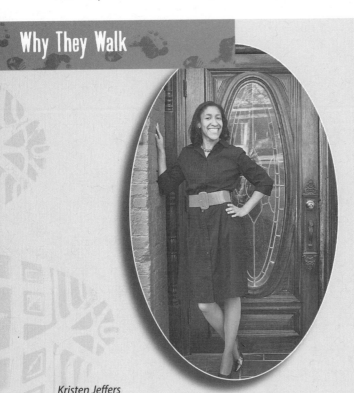

Kristen Jeffers

*I walk first and foremost because I have two feet and two legs that work. So many people worldwide don't even have that, and I try to make it a habit to count my most basic blessings. A cousin of mine walked with his family down to the ocean one August afternoon almost two years ago. Yet, unlike the rest of our family, he was not able to walk back to shore. A swimming accident has left him gradually trying to regain strength in all of his extremities. Walking is only a goal, a distant dream right now. He has not given up, but it makes me think about how the simple act of using one's two feet and two legs to propel oneself could be snatched away at any moment.*

*When we use the word walkability in the professional planning sector, there is a focus on what able-bodied people can or cannot do.*

We also only focus on what I would call "choice" walkers, people who drive to a "town center" district or their original central business district, now revived, to take in a play at the regional theater, drink and be merry at the local microbrewery, or plan the next revolution at the local coffeehouse.

While we are holding our cup of coffee, talking about how to fix poverty, poverty walks right by that window all day long. Poverty can't afford a car. Actually, poverty used to have a car until he wrecked it after a fight with a friend. Poverty was also paralyzed just like my cousin, but he gradually regained strength — seemingly miraculously, but helped because he was once a state government employee with good health insurance that allowed him the hospital stay he needed. Poverty's also young enough that he's not ready to sit down and his brain is quite lucid. He knows his way around a tool shed and literally can bring light to dark rooms, from his years of training and working as a licensed electrician. Poverty's also the reason I'm here, because poverty's known to me as Dad.

When I was little, Dad was determined that I would know how to read a map and know how to get myself around. When I was little, that consisted of walking the streets of our neighborhood. Our neighborhood was built in the first wave of suburban construction after World War II. It was all white at one point, despite being home to both single-family, owner-occupied homes and a housing project. A colleague of mine had a parent who grew up there in those days. I grew up in the days when pizza delivery was nonexistent, drugs were rampant, and most of the faces on my block were as brown as my own. Yet, as I walked or later biked down the street, many of those neighbors looked out for me and made my trips very exciting and fun.

It's those memories that I draw from when I walk and bike today. I know what it's like to bike and walk for fun. I know what it's like to walk and bike because that's your only choice. I fortunately do *not know what it's like to not have that choice. Yet, all three of these make me continue to be involved in the movement for complete streets. Sure, my dad or I could walk through unmarked grassy areas next to a four-lane road, but can my cousin do that? Is it really safe to be only inches from sixty-mile-an-hour traffic? My hope is that now that I'm in a position of privilege, with a driver's license, a working, fuel-efficient car and an office just a fifteen-minute walk away from my newish luxury apartment, I can tell others that it's not just people like my dad who walk. Everyone with an able body can walk. And if they have smaller wheels than a car, then there's room on the sidewalk for them, too.*

— Kristen Jeffers
Raleigh, NC

I hope this book has inspired you, made you laugh and, most importantly, moved you to action. People often say to me, "It all sounds great, but how can I do that? How can I walk during the day where I live, when I don't live in Savannah or some other walkable place?" Fortunately, no matter where we live, there's a lot each of us can do. Here are a few possibilities:

1. **Walk more — now.**
   It really is that easy. If you live someplace where you have destinations you can walk to within a ten- or fifteen-minute walk, start doing so daily. If you live somewhere where things are farther away, at least start walking more for recreation. Get in the habit. Walk a mile a day at first, which takes the average person about twenty minutes. Eventually make that walk two miles per day. Make the effort to walk to shops, parks, friends' houses or other nearby destinations. Force yourself to do things others might think is strange, such as

walking across parking lots at large strip malls. Walking is great for your health even if it's just for recreation, so start doing it today. And support those local businesses that make life easier for walkers. People often say, "Oh, but I commute," or "Oh, but I have kids to cart around all day." Don't succumb to Oh-buts. There's always a reason to say "I can't." But life is far more interesting when we learn to say "I can."

2. *Bike more — now.*
Bikes are cheap, and they're fun. Remember learning how to ride a bike as a kid? It really is as easy as jumping back on. It's amazing how quickly that sensation of fun comes back when you're on two wheels. Even better, the bike allows you to get to a lot of destinations that are farther away. So if you live somewhere that makes walking to places difficult, try the bike. Ride on the sidewalk if you have to in order to build confidence. Do whatever it takes to get used to that feeling again. But please — don't buy Spandex!

3. *Encourage others to walk and bike, especially young people.*
Now that you've gotten yourself going, encourage others to try it, too. Talk with your family, your friends, and that kid next door. Become a positive, but not annoying, example to everyone else. Getting kids going is so important, since good and bad habits start early. As the saying goes, be the change you want to see.

4. *Move, if you're able to.*
That's right, I'm telling you to pack up and relocate. It's not as difficult as you think. I moved halfway across the country to a place where I knew almost no one. You can certainly move across town to a neighborhood that is better for walking. Take the chance, and you'll never look back. We ultimately vote with our feet, so find that great place and go.

## 5. *Make your voice heard.*

Finally, make your voice heard for better walking and biking infrastructure, zoning reform and better buildings. I don't expect everyone to be as passionate about this as I am. But once the bug hits, you may find that you want to do more. That's great: your community needs you and your passion. More than anything, our cities need people who can speak up for better sidewalks, better-protected bike lanes, slower traffic speeds, and so much more. We have decades of bad ideas to undo, from building too much parking to ramming freeways through cities. Some of your time can be spent on small and quick efforts — look up *Tactical Urbanism* and *Build a Better Block* for examples. Other civic efforts may take years of your

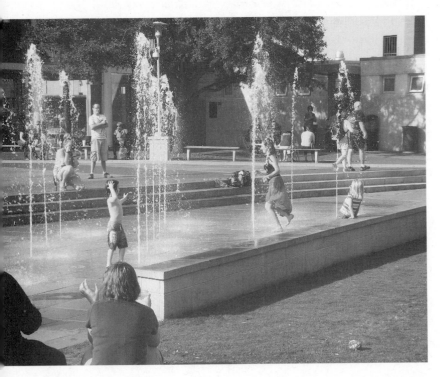

*Kids love walkable places.*

time to push back against the car culture that has been a cancer on our neighborhoods for far too long. We need you. Make your presence felt.

For my part, I simply plan to keep walking and keep working on making walking easier for others. The changes I've made in my life have enriched it far more than I could have imagined, and my hope is that more people can enjoy the same benefits. This life that is lived outdoors more often, using my own body to get around, feels very natural and, well, *human*. At forty-three, I feel as healthy and happy as I ever have, and am living a lifestyle that I've wanted for many years.

But tomorrow is Tuesday, and it's time to get ready for the day. Just another ordinary Tuesday, with places to go, people to see — and walks to take.

## Why They Walk

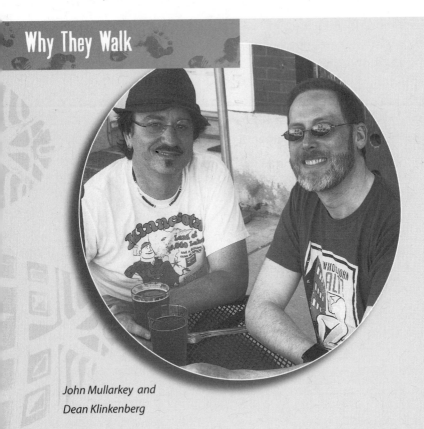

John Mullarkey and
Dean Klinkenberg

We live in an old city neighborhood, old for the US, anyway. My partner and I chose to live in this neighborhood because of the variety of places we can get to on foot. From our house, we can walk to one of the best botanical gardens in the world; to a lovely, Victorian-inspired park; and to a thriving business district where we can eat Thai, Vietnamese, Italian, classic American or Ethiopian food or grab a drink at a corner bar, a dance bar or a dive bar. Sometimes we walk to these places because we want the exercise. Sometimes we walk to avoid fighting confused suburbanites for a parking spot. Usually we walk just because we can.

On a typical walk, we may hear the squeak of sneakers on concrete, the ping of a softball propelled by an aluminum bat, maybe *someone yelling "Goal!" We slow our pace to admire the intricate masonry designs executed by nineteenth-century immigrants to St. Louis who sculpted patterns with bricks fired a couple of miles away. We stop to talk to neighbors and friends. We walk because it reminds us where we are.*

— Dean Klinkenberg and John Mullarkey

St. Louis, MO

# Index

*The Rise of the Creative Class,* 30
road safety, 91, 99
Rodgers Forge, 137–138
routes, variety of, 66, 68–69, 70–71, 88
running, 12, 69–70, 86, 88–89

safety, 59–61, 81, 88, 99, 145. *See also* road safety.
Savannah, walkability, 4, 13, 50, 69, 88, 106, 129
schools, 32, 58, 59, 61, 99, 137, 145
Sease, Tony, 44–46
sharing economy, 53–54. *See also* bikeshares.
shoes, 116
shopping options, 144–145
Sirota, Stuart, 136–138
sitting, 83
snow days, 72–73
socializing, and walking, 104–135
Sobel, Lee, 16–17
St. Louis, 37
street closures, 70–72
stress, 27-28, 90–92

three-mile-per-hour city, 113
Tomasulo, Matt, 80–82
tourist hotspots, in US, 134
traffic calming, 82
trains, 16, 55, 56
transportation, spending on, 18.
    *See also* car ownership.
trash, 129, 131–132

vacations, and walking, 133–135
violence, and children, 58–59
*virtuous circle,* 24

## About the Author

Kevin Klinkenberg is the Principal Designer at K2 Urban Design. For more than two decades he has been working to create sustainable, sociable environments and walkable communities in cooperation with developers, cities and nonprofits. A huge fan of the sharing economy, Kevin recently established the car sharing company, Share Savannah, to help his neighbors realize their goals of living car-free or "car-light." He believes that the 21st century is a time to reclaim our lost 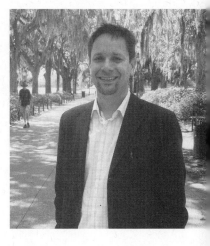 traditions, connect better with each other and use our advanced technologies in ways that are much more human.

Kevin blogs at www.kevinklinkenberg.com

If you have enjoyed *Why I Walk*, you might also enjoy other

# BOOKS TO BUILD A NEW SOCIETY

Our books provide positive solutions for people who want to make a difference. We specialize in:

**Sustainable Living • Green Building • Peak Oil
Renewable Energy • Environment & Economy Natural
Building & Appropriate Technology Progressive Leadership
• Resistance and Community Educational & Parenting Resources**

---

## New Society Publishers

### ENVIRONMENTAL BENEFITS STATEMENT

New Society Publishers has chosen to produce this book on recycled paper made with **100% post consumer waste,** processed chlorine free, and old growth free.

For every 5,000 books printed, New Society saves the following resources:[1]

| | |
|---|---|
| 16 | Trees |
| 1,462 | Pounds of Solid Waste |
| 1,609 | Gallons of Water |
| 2,089 | Kilowatt Hours of Electricity |
| 2,658 | Pounds of Greenhouse Gases |
| 11 | Pounds of HAPs, VOCs, and AOX Combined |
| 4 | Cubic Yards of Landfill Space |

[1]Environmental benefits are calculated based on research done by the Environmental Defense Fund and other members of the Paper Task Force who study the environmental impacts of the paper industry.

---

*For a full list of NSP's titles, please call* 1-800-567-6772 *or check out our website* at:

**www.newsociety.com**

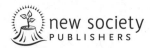

new society
PUBLISHERS